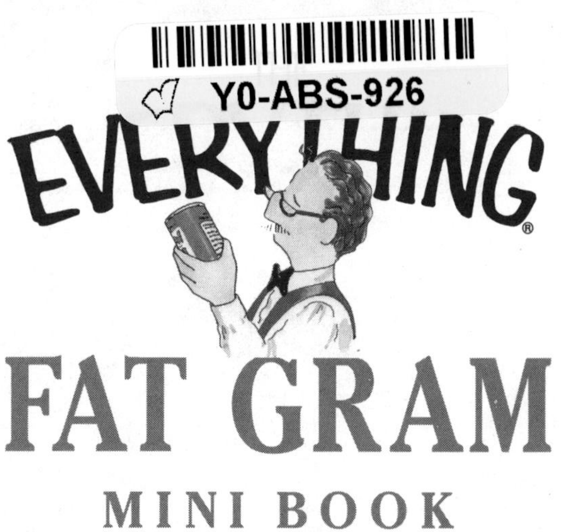

THE EVERYTHING® FAT GRAM MINI BOOK

Barbara Ravage

Adams Media Corporation
Avon, Massachusetts

An Everything® Series Book.
"Everything" is a registered trademark of Adams Media Corporation.

Published by Adams Media Corporation
57 Littlefield Street, Avon, MA 02322
www.adamsmedia.com

ISBN: 1-58062-608-4

Printed in Canada.

J I H G F E D C B A

Library of Congress Cataloging-in-Publication Data
available from the publisher.

Cover illustrations by Barry Littmann.
Interior illustrations by Barry Littmann.
Additional contributions by Susan Gaber.

Contents

Introduction

The Everything® Fat Gram Mini Book is designed as a compact reference, small enough to slip into your pocket or purse when you go to the supermarket or are eating away from home. It won't take up much space on your kitchen counter either, so you can refer to it when you are planning and preparing meals.

How to Use This Book

This book contains the fat content in grams of over 3,000 foods and ingredients, organized in

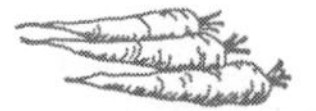

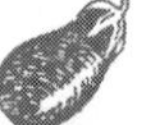

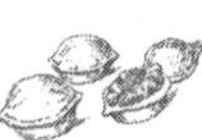
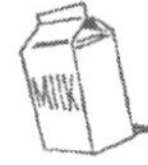

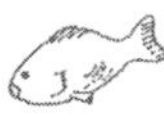
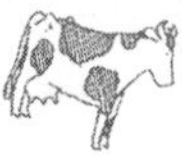

categories to make it easy to find what you're looking for. The main categories, arranged in alphabetical order, are:

1. Beverages, including alcoholic and soft drinks, as well as fruit and vegetable juices
2. Breads, crackers, and baked goods
3. Cereals, grains, rice, and pasta
4. Dairy and eggs, including milk and milk beverages
5. Diet and health foods
6. Extras, including dressings, gravies, sauces, condiments, flavorings, herbs, and spices
7. Fats and oils
8. Fish and seafood
9. Fruits
10. Meats and poultry
11. Nuts and seeds
12. Snack foods

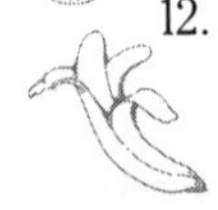
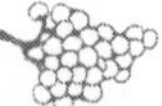

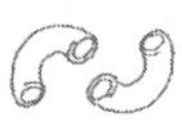 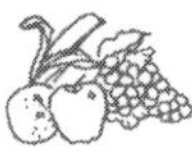 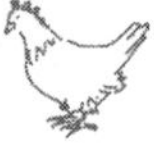 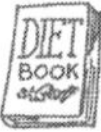

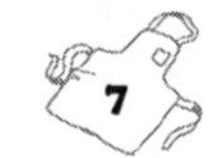

13. Soup, stews, casseroles, and other combination foods
14. Sweets and desserts, including common baking ingredients
15. Vegetables and dried beans

How to Find What You're Looking For

Within each category, foods are arranged by subcategories. For example, within "Meats and Poultry," you will find beef, pork, lamb, chicken, duck, turkey, and so on. And within those subcategories, you will find specific cuts of meat or poultry and methods of preparation.

In an effort to include as many foods as possible, branded items have been listed only when they are unique and cannot be covered by a general item. For example, Cola is listed among soft

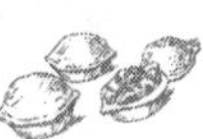
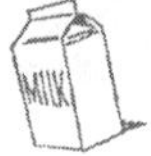

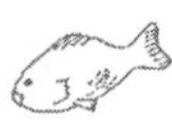
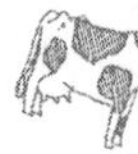

drinks, but Dr. Pepper is listed by brand name. General listings are often averages of several brand-name items. For example, there are many different brands of yogurt and many give different names to their flavors: french vanilla or vanilla, mixed fruit or fruit medley, etc. Instead of listing them all, yogurts are distinguished by their fat content (whole milk, low fat, and no fat) and an average fat gram count is used.

In all of these cases, if you are looking for an exact fat gram count, look at the label on the product in question.

What You Won't Find

Because there are literally tens of thousands of different food products on supermarket shelves, no attempt has been made to list every item and every brand. In particular, special diet foods that

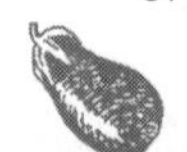
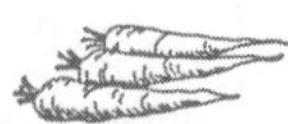

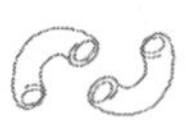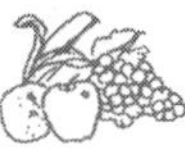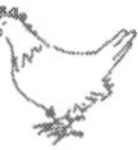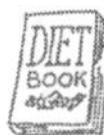

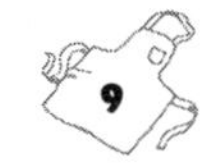

are available in supermarkets as well as from weight-loss programs are too numerous to mention. Nonetheless, all of these items are labeled with their fat content in grams, allowing you to figure out how much fat you are consuming.

What Is Fat?

Fats, also called lipids, are molecules that occur naturally in many plants and animals. Oils are pure fats in liquid form that are extracted from plant and animal sources.

The fats we eat are called *dietary fats.* They are used by the body in many different ways:

- They supply immediate energy or can be stored for use at another time.
- They are an important part of many body cells.

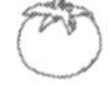
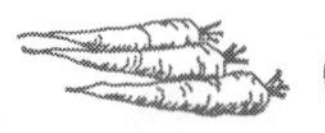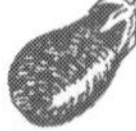

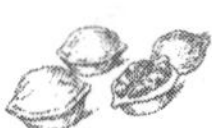
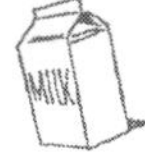

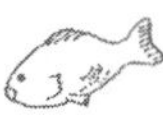
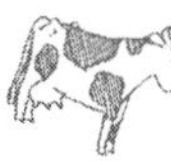

- They transport nutrients, including many vitamins.
- They contribute to normal growth and development.

There are several different kinds of dietary fat:

- **Saturated fat,** which is solid at room temperature, comes mostly from animal sources. This includes butter and lard, and the fat you see in (marbling) and around a piece of steak or a pork chop, for example.
- **Unsaturated fat,** which is liquid at room temperature, comes from plant sources. Vegetable oils, including corn and olive oil, are unsaturated fats. There are two exceptions to this rule: Coconut and palm (or palm kernel) oils are saturated fats, even though they come from plants. If you are watching your fat intake, pay attention to this

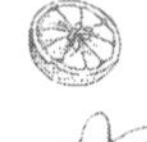
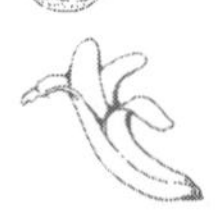
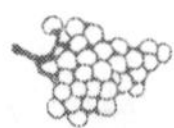

> since many commercial baked goods—cookies, crackers, and the like—are made with coconut or palm oil or both.

There are several types of unsaturated fat: monounsaturated and polyunsaturated are the two main types.

All fats have an effect on the amount of cholesterol in your blood. Saturated fats raise the level of low-density lipoprotein, or LDL, commonly known as the "bad cholesterol." Unsaturated fats do not raise LDL levels; in fact, they seem to lower them.

Trans Fats

There is another kind of fat, a kind of Frankenstein monster that comes from unsaturated fat but has the bad qualities of saturated fat. This manufactured

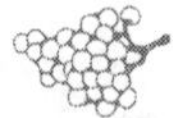

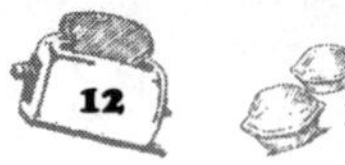

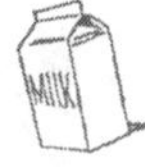
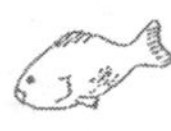

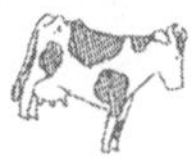

molecule is made by adding extra hydrogen atoms to unsaturated fat molecules. That's why these fats are called *hydrogenated,* a term you may have seen on some food labels.

Hydrogenated fats are all *trans fats,* that is, they have been transformed so that a formerly liquid fat takes a solid form at room temperature.

Hydrogenation is the secret to margarine, in fact, which has a solid form even though it is an unsaturated fat. That means margarine is a major source of trans fats, which makes any claims about it being more "heart healthy" than butter highly questionable. In fact, studies have shown that people whose diets are high in trans fats are at increased risk for heart attack.

Hydrogenation also keeps fats from becoming rancid, so it is used in many baked goods and other foods that are stored without

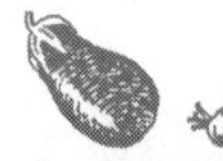
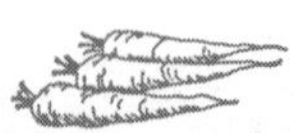

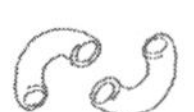 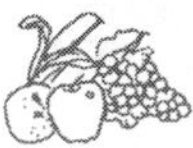 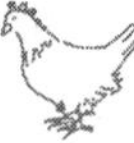 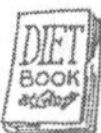

refrigeration. Cookies and crackers often contain trans fats.

Although it is a good idea to avoid trans fats as much as possible, doing so is difficult. According to current food labeling laws, the word "trans fat" does not have to be used. These regulations may be changing, but for now trans fats are truly "stealth fats."

There is a way to do some sleuthing, however. One way is to look for the words "hydrogenated" and "partially hydrogenated" on the label of all prepared foods you buy and try to avoid these foods as much as you can.

Why Limit Fat?

Regardless of type, every gram of fat contains 9 calories. This is in contrast to 4 calories per

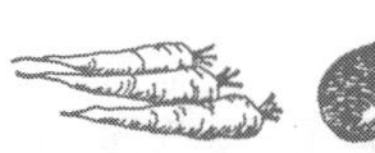

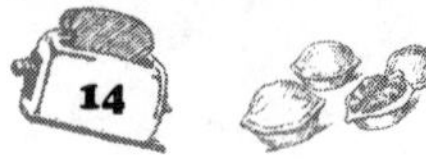

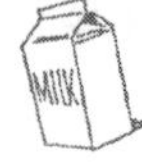

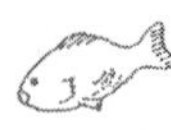
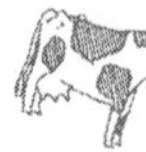

gram each for proteins and carbohydrates. (Remember that 28 grams equals 1 ounce.)

Dietary fat is not only high in calories, it also contributes to many health problems. These include heart disease, high blood pressure, and diabetes. Although it has not been proven, many types of cancer seem to occur more often in people who eat a lot of fat.

People trying to lose weight can cut their calorie intake by more than half by substituting carbohydrates and protein for fat. That is, fat contains more than twice as many calories as these other nutrients. People who have been told by a doctor to limit fat intake for other health reasons may avoid health problems or improve their conditions by following a low-fat diet.

Doing that is easier said than done, however, since few foods contain only a single nutrient

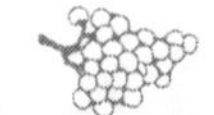

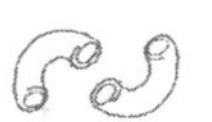  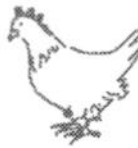 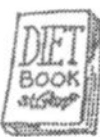 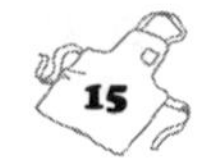

type. Most are combinations, which is why you need a fat gram counter such as this one.

How Much Fat Do You Need?

Everyone needs some fat in the diet, but how much is still not certain. According to some experts, fats should make up no more than 30 percent of a person's daily caloric intake. Others say it should be an even smaller percentage, going as low as 10 percent.

Given the way most of us eat, there is little danger of having a fat-deficient diet. The challenge is to eat a well-rounded diet that has the proper proportion of fat.

One way to figure this out is to take your weight and divide by two. That equals approximately the number of grams of fat you should eat each day, assuming the middle ground of

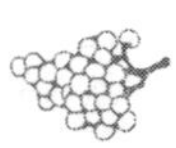

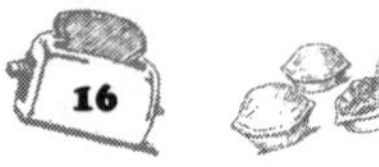

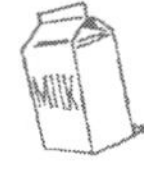
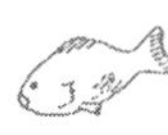

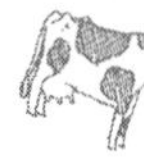

20 percent. For example, if you weigh 160 pounds, you should have no more than 80 grams of fat each day.

Losing Weight by Limiting Fat

Losing weight is a complicated matter. Theoretically, you can do it by reducing calorie intake over a period of time at the rate of 3,500 calories per pound you wish to lose. That's because each pound of stored fat represents 3,500 calories. If you eat 3,500 more calories than your body needs, you will gain a pound. If you eat 3,500 fewer calories than your body needs, you will lose a pound. It is far more effective, realistic, and long-lasting to reduce calorie intake *and* increase level of activity. That way, you take in fewer calories and burn more through exercise. Not only will you lose weight,

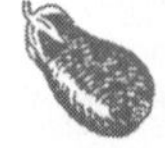
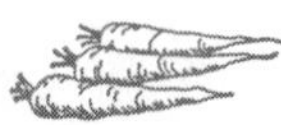

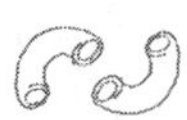 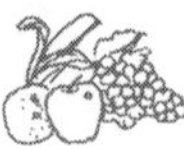 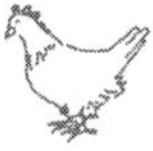 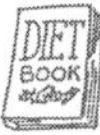

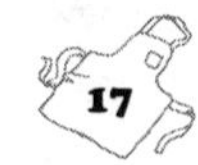

you will also look and feel better, and improve your overall health.

Still, limiting fat gives you more bang for your buck since each gram of fat contains 9 calories compared to 4 calories each for proteins and carbohydrates. That's where low-fat foods come in.

Many foods are labeled low or reduced fat, but others are naturally low in fats. Most fruits and practically all vegetables have little or no fat at all. If you have a sweet tooth, carbonated soft drinks, juices, sugars, syrups, jams, jellies, and many kinds of candy are free of fat. They may be high in calories, but they get them from sugar, a carbohydrate.

Alcohol also contains no fat, so most alcoholic beverages are low or no fat items. That doesn't make them healthful choices, however. Alcohol contains almost as many calories as fat:

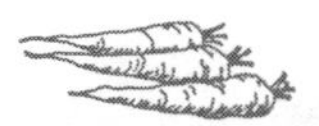 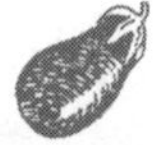

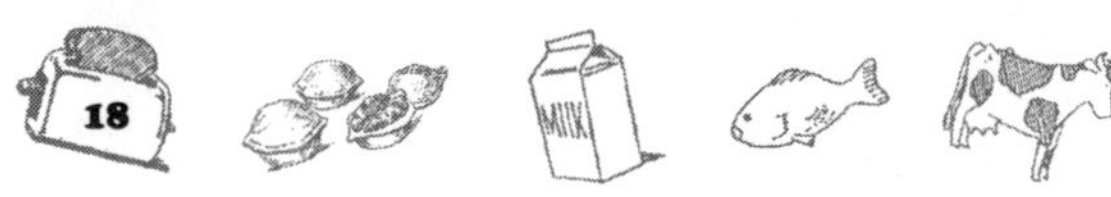

7 per gram. That makes drinking alcoholic beverages a poor way to reduce calories. In addition, many other health and social problems are associated with excess alcohol consumption.

The best way to limit fats is to increase the amount of fruits and vegetables you eat. Not only are they low or no fat foods, they tend to be high-bulk foods as well. That is, they take up a lot of room on the plate (so they look like a lot of food) and in your stomach (so they help you feel full).

What Is a Serving?

Serving (or portion) size is an amount set by the Food and Drug Administration that corresponds to how much an average person would eat. All food labels are required by law to indicate the number of grams of fat per serving, not per package or

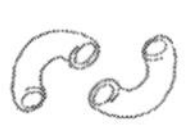  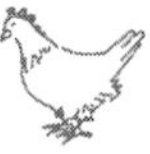 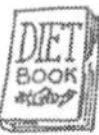 

container. For people who are counting fat grams, *this is a very important point.*

A box of crackers contains more than one serving. If you imagine that the per-serving fat gram count refers to the entire box, you will be in for a nasty surprise the next time you get on the scale or have your blood cholesterol tested. Likewise, many canned or bottled beverages contain more than a single serving. Moreover, muffins, bagels, and other baked goods vary in size and therefore fat content.

The best thing to do is to read labels, if possible, and do some number crunching on your own. The only way to be sure you are consuming the number of grams of fat you think you are is to pay attention to serving size.

You can measure servings in various ways. Sometimes it is a matter of counting pieces. Other times a measuring cup, spoon, or kitchen

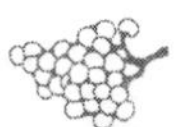

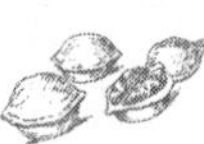
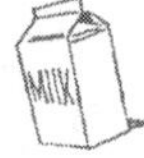

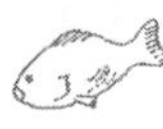
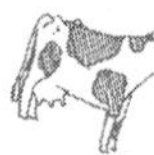

scale will give you the information you need. For packaged food, it may be a matter of dividing the contents into the number of servings it contains, and eating only one portion.

After a while, you will have a pretty good idea of what a serving of a particular food looks like. Still, it is a good idea to start out by measuring. Go back to measuring every once in a while to maintain accuracy. "Portion creep" is a major contributing factor to the failure of weight-loss plans and fat-reduction diets, and the problems of obesity and heart disease in general.

Read the Label!

According to the law, all packaged and prepared foods must carry nutritional information, including fat content, on their labels. This

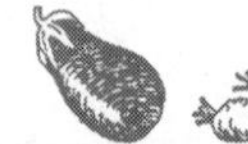
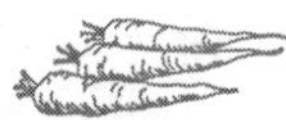

includes foods that come in boxes, cans, bottles, and numerous other containers. Fresh fruits and vegetables, unprocessed meats, and other "unpackaged" foods are not included. Nonetheless, most of the foods Americans buy and eat are covered by the label law. Reading labels can give you a lot of useful information, if you know how to look for it.

- **Serving size** is perhaps the most important piece of information you will find on a label. Except for single-serving items, food packages contain more than one serving. The first two lines on the approved food label tell you the size of a serving and the number of servings in the package.
- **Calorie content** is the next important piece of data. The number of calories indicated is always *per serving,* not per package. You can determine the number of calories in the whole

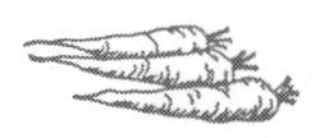 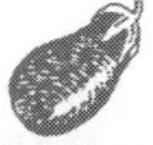

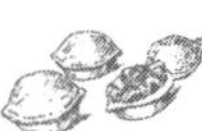
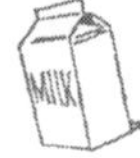

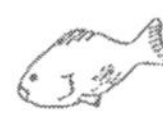
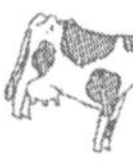

package by multiplying calories by number of servings. That's a good way to find out how many calories you are actually getting if you eat (or drink) "the whole thing"!

- For people who are counting fat grams, the label provides a lot of information. It lists the number of *calories from fat* and the *percent of the daily value*. That percent is based on a theoretical typical person, so it is only a general guide.
- More important, the label also lists the *per serving fat content by gram* of all the fat, and also breaks out saturated fat. Monounsaturated, polyunsaturated, and trans fats are not singled out according to regulations now in effect.
- **Ingredients** are listed in order of their weight. That is, the earlier in the list an ingredient appears, the more (by weight) there is of it. This is where manufacturers may try to pull the wool

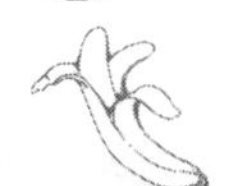
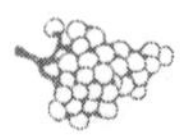

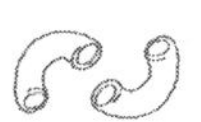  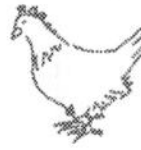 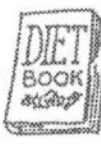 

over your eyes. But if you know their tricks, you won't be fooled.

The two areas where the label writers can fudge are sugar and fats, especially those stealthy trans fats. If you look for any words that say "fat" to you, and you find them close to the bottom of the list, you might think there isn't much fat in that particular food. In fact, fat goes by many names, and most packaged foods contain more than one type. A single food might contain butter, lard, hydrogenated and partially hydrogenated vegetable oils (that's where your trans fats are), fish oils, shortening, and any number of fat-containing ingredients, such as lecithin, milk, eggs, and more. Small amounts (by weight) of many different fats can be used to hide the true story of the fat content. The way to unmask these ingredients is to look back at the total fat grams part of the label.

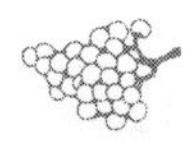

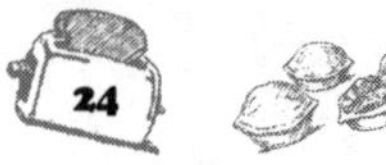
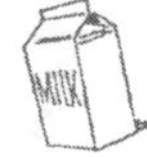
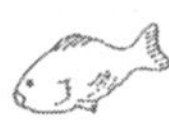
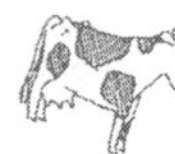

Decoding Labeling Terms

Diet- and health-conscious people may look for the terms *low fat, reduced fat, no fat, low calorie, reduced calorie,* and *light (or lite)* when they are making food selections. But what do these terms mean? The short answer is that they do not necessarily mean a food is low in calories and/or fat. The long answer comes from the federal Food and Drug Administration (FDA), which has set strict rules about the use of these terms:

- *Free* means that a product contains no amount of, or only trivial amounts of, fat, saturated fat, cholesterol, sodium, sugars, and/or calories.
- *Low (or Lo)* means the food can be eaten frequently without exceeding dietary guidelines for fat, saturated fat, cholesterol,

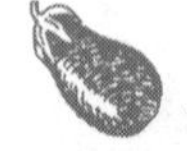
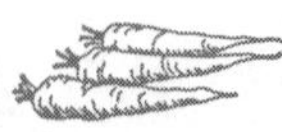

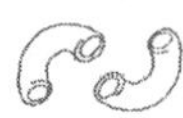
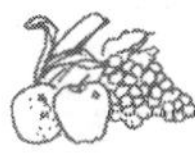
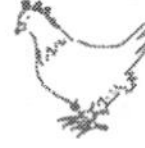
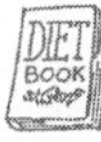

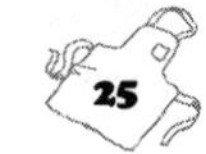

sodium, and/or calories. According to this definition, low calorie means 40 calories or less per serving; low fat means 3 grams of fat or less per serving.

- *Reduced* means that the product contains at least 25 percent less fat or calories than the regular product. However, a reduced claim can't be made on a product if the regular version meets the requirement for a "low" claim. For example, all pretzels are low in fat, so a particular brand of pretzels cannot be termed "reduced fat." And although they are a good snack alternative to potato chips for people who are watching their fat intake, they are not a low-calorie item. Pretzels get their calories from carbohydrates, at the rate of 4 calories per gram.
- *Less* means that a food contains 25 percent less of fat or calories than the regular version.

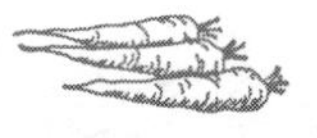

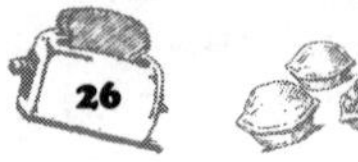

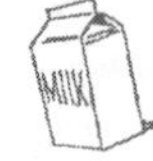
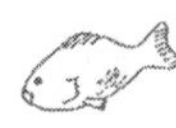

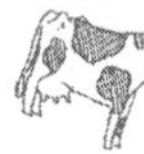

For example, pretzels that have 25 percent less fat than potato chips could carry a "less" claim.

- *Light (or Lite)* can means that a product contains one-third fewer calories or half the fat of the regular version. If the food derives 50 percent or more of its calories from fat, the reduction must be 50 percent of the fat.

Be aware, though, that "light" can also be used to refer to salt (sodium) content and to describe such properties as texture and color, as long as the label explains the intent—"light brown sugar" and "light and fluffy."

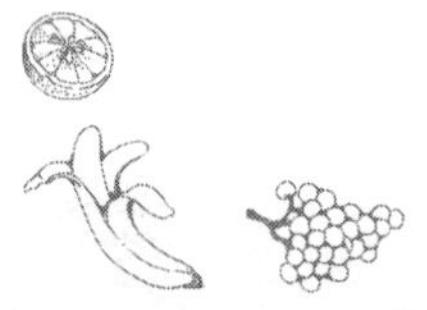

Food	Serving Size	Fat
Alcoholic Beverages		
ale	12 oz	0
beer		
regular	12 oz	0
light	12 oz	0
low-alcohol (2.3% alcohol)	12 oz	0
non-alcoholic (less than .5% alcohol)	12 oz	0
malt liquor	12 oz	0
cider (6% alcohol)	12 oz	0
cocktails, mixed drinks		
bloody mary	5 oz	tr
brandy alexander	3 oz	15
daiquiri	2 oz	tr
egg nog	3 oz	19
gimlet	3 oz	0
gin and tonic	6 oz	0
Irish coffee	6 oz	9
manhattan	2 oz	0
margarita	3½ oz	0
martini (gin or vodka)	2 oz	0
mint julep	4½ oz	2.5
piña colada	4½ oz	2.5
scotch and soda	4 oz	0
screwdriver	7 oz	0
tequila sunrise	6 oz	tr
tom collins	7½ oz	0
vodka and tonic (see *gin and tonic*)		
whiskey sour	3 oz	tr

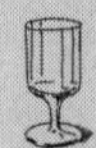

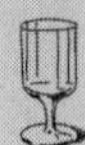

Food	Serving Size	Fat
Alcoholic Beverages *(continued)*		
cocktails, mixed drinks *(continued)*		
wine spritzer	6 oz	0
dessert wine		
madeira	2 oz	0
marsala	2 oz	0
port	2 oz	0
sherry, dry	2 oz	0
sherry, sweet	2 oz	0
vermouth, dry	2 oz	0
vermouth, sweet	2 oz	0
liqueurs		
amaretto	1 oz	0
brandy, fruit	1 oz	0
Benedictine	1 oz	0
Irish cream	1 oz	0
Cointreau	1 oz	0
coffee	1 oz	0
crème de cacao	1 oz	0
crème de menthe	1 oz	0
Drambuie	1 oz	0
Grand Marnier	1 oz	0
kirsch	1 oz	0
ouzo	1 oz	0
pastis	1 oz	0
Sambuca	1 oz	0
Southern Comfort	1 oz	0
triple sec	1 oz	0

Food	Serving Size	Fat

Alcoholic Beverages *(continued)*

liquors: bourbon, brandy, gin, rum, scotch, tequila, vodka, whisky		
80 proof	1 oz	0
86 proof	1 oz	0
90 proof	1 oz	0
100 proof	1 oz	0
table wine		
champagne	4 oz	0
red	4 oz	0
rose	4 oz	0
white, dry	4 oz	0
white, sweet	4 oz	0

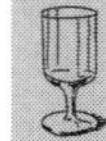

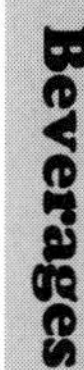

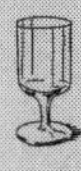

Breakfast Drinks*

chocolate		
powder	individual packet	1
sugar free	individual packet	1
strawberry		
powder	individual packet	tr
sugar free	individual packet	0
vanilla		
powder	individual packet	0
sugar free	individual packet	0
ready to drink (all flavors)	10 oz	3

*Average fat; fat counts vary widely among brands.

Food	Serving Size	Fat
Chocolate Beverages*		
chocolate drink, bottled	8 oz	1
cocoa, hot chocolate		
with whole milk	8 oz	10
with nonfat milk	8 oz	2
cocoa, hot chocolate mix		
with whole milk	8 oz	8.75
with 2% milk	8 oz	5.75
with water	8 oz	1.25
artificially sweetened	8 oz	.5
Coffee		
black		
regular or decaffeinated brewed or instant	8 oz	0
café au lait		
with whole milk	8 oz	3.5
with nonfat milk	8 oz	.5
caffe latte		
with whole milk	8 oz	3.5
with nonfat milk	8 oz	.5
cappuccino		
with whole milk	8 oz	3.5
with nonfat milk	8 oz	0

*Average fat; fat counts vary widely among brands.

Food	Serving Size	Fat
Coffee *(continued)*		
espresso	2 oz	0
flavored*		
made with water	8 oz	3
sugar free	8 oz	1.5
substitute, grain beverage	8 oz	0
Fruit Juices and Blends		
apple		
juice, cider	8 oz	.25
blended juice drink	8 oz	.25
cranberry, cocktail		
regular	8 oz	.25
low-cal	8 oz	0
cranberry-apple	8 oz	0
cranberry-grape	8 oz	.25
fruit punch		
canned	8 oz	0
made from frozen concentrate	8 oz	0
made from powder	8 oz	0

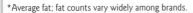

*Average fat; fat counts vary widely among brands.

Food	Serving Size	Fat
Fruit Juices and Blends *(continued)*		
grape		
canned/bottled	8 oz	.25
juice drink, canned	8 oz	0
grapefruit		
fresh, canned, unsweetened	8 oz	.25
sweetened	8 oz	.25
frozen	8 oz	0
lemon		
fresh	1 tbsp	0
	1 cup	0
concentrate	1 tbsp	0
	1 cup	0
lemonade		
made from frozen concentrate	8 oz	0
made from powder	8 oz	0
sugar free	8 oz	0
lime *(see lemon)*		
limeade		
made from frozen concentrate	8 oz	0
nectars: apricot, peach, pear, papaya	8 oz	.25
orange		
juice, canned, fresh, frozen	8 oz	.5
blended drink	8 oz	0

Food	Serving Size	Fat
Fruit Juices and Blends *(continued)*		
orange *(continued)*		
powdered drink	8 oz	0
sugar free	8 oz	0
orange-grapefruit	8 oz	0.25
pineapple, canned, frozen	8 oz	tr
pineapple-grapefruit	8 oz	.25
prune	8 oz	0
smoothies*		
fruit	8 oz	0
fruit and milk	8 oz	.5
fruit and yogurt	8 oz	.5
nutritional shakes *(see Diet and Health Foods)*		
Shakes		
chocolate	12 oz	12.5
malted	12 oz	13.75
vanilla	12 oz	10
malted	12 oz	11.75

*Average fat; fat counts vary widely among brands. Fat counts are based on an 8-oz serving; many containers hold more than one serving, so read the label.

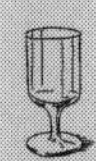

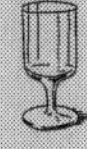

Food	Serving Size	Fat
Sodas and Soft Drinks		
bitter lemon	8 oz	0
cherry	8 oz	0
citrus	8 oz	0
club	8 oz	0
cola		
regular	8 oz	0
cherry	8 oz	0
collins mixer	8 oz	0
cream	8 oz	0
diet (all brands, all flavors)	8 oz	0
Dr. Pepper	8 oz	0
ginger ale	8 oz	0
cherry	8 oz	0
grape	8 oz	0
lemon/lime	8 oz	0
mineral water		
plain	8 oz	0
flavored	8 oz	0

Food	Serving Size	Fat

Sodas and Soft Drinks *(continued)*

Food	Serving Size	Fat
orange	8 oz	0
piña colada	8 oz	0
quinine water (see *tonic*)		
root beer	8 oz	0
seltzer		
plain	8 oz	0
flavored	8 oz	0
Seven-Up	8 oz	0
tonic	8 oz	0
vanilla	8 oz	0

Sports Drinks

There are many brands of "sports" and "energy" drinks and they come in various sizes. The nutritional content varies widely among brands. Read the label of any drink you use and pay particular attention to the serving size as a bottle may contain more than one serving.

Tea

Food	Serving Size	Fat
regular or decaffeinated (brewed or instant, unsweetened)	8 oz	0
flavored	8 oz	0

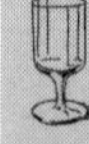
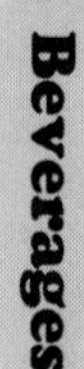

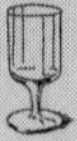

Food	Serving Size	Fat
Tea *(continued)*		
herbal	8 oz	0
iced		
unsweetened	8 oz	0
from powdered mix	8 oz	0
bottled, canned	8 oz	0
Vegetable Juices		
bloody mary mix	8 oz	0
carrot	8 oz	.5
tomato	8 oz	0
tomato beef	8 oz	0
tomato clam	8 oz	0
tomato-vegetable blend	8 oz	0

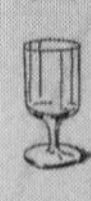

Food	Serving Size	Fat
Bread*		
bran	1 oz slice	2
challah	1 oz slice	2
corn (see *Muffins, Sweet Rolls, Sweet Breads)*		
cracked wheat	1 oz slice	1
focaccia (see *Pizza)*		
French	2 oz slice	2.25
honey-wheat berry	1 oz slice	1
Irish soda	1 oz slice	3
Italian	2 oz slice	2.25
multigrain	1 oz slice	1.5
oat bran	1 oz slice	1
oatmeal	1 oz slice	1.25
pita	1	.75
whole wheat	1	1.75
potato	1 oz slice	2

*Average fat; fat counts vary widely among brands as does weight of slices.

Food	Serving Size	Fat
Bread *(continued)*		
pumpernickel	1 oz slice	.75
raisin	1 oz slice	1.75
rye	1 oz slice	1
sourdough	2 oz slice	2
white, sandwich style	1 slice	1
	thin slice (.6 oz)	.5
whole wheat	1 slice	1
bread crumbs	1 cup	5.75
breadsticks	1 piece	1
croutons	1 cup	2
stuffing, dry	1 cup	17
Buns, Rolls, and Biscuits*		
bagel		
plain, onion, seeded	small, 2 oz	1.5
	medium, 3 oz	2
	large, 4 oz	3
cinnamon raisin	medium, 3 oz	10
egg	medium, 3 oz	8

*Average fat; fat counts vary widely among brands and recipes.

Food	Serving Size	Fat
Buns, Rolls, and Biscuits *(continued)*		
biscuit		
baking powder	1 oz	5
buttermilk	1 oz	4
crescent	1 oz	5.5
croissant	2 oz	12
dinner	1 oz	2
english muffin		
plain	1	1
whole wheat	1	1.5
cinnamon raisin	1	1.75
sandwich size	1	1.75
French	1	1.5
hamburger	1	2.25
hoagie	1	1.75
hot dog	1	2
Italian	1	3.5
kaiser, with poppy seeds	1	2
sandwich, with sesame seeds	1	4

Food	Serving Size	Fat
Crackers*		
animal	11 pieces	3.5
cheese		
peanut butter sandwich	1 piece	1.5
mini	14 pieces	8
corn cakes	2 cakes	.25
crispbread	1 piece	tr
goldfish	55 pieces	3
graham	1 oz; 4 squares	3
low fat	1 oz; 4 squares	1.5
melba toast	1 piece	tr
matzo	1 square	.5
oat thins	18 crackers	6
oyster	23 crackers	1.5
rice cakes	1 piece	.5
saltine	1 piece	.5
fat free	1 piece	0
sesame	3 pieces	1

*Average fat; fat counts vary widely among brands.

Food	Serving Size	Fat
Crackers *(continued)*		
shredded wheat	7 pieces	5
reduced fat	8 pieces	3
snack rounds	5 pieces	4
minis	48 pieces	9
soda	2 pieces	1.5
stone ground wheat	5 pieces	3
vegetable thins	14 pieces	9
water	5 pieces	2
wheat	5 pieces	1
wheat thins	16 pieces	6
reduced fat	18 pieces	4
zwieback	1 piece	1
Muffins and Quick Breads*		
banana nut		
bread	1 oz slice	6.5
muffin	2½" × 2¼" slice	5
toaster muffin	1.4 oz	5.75

*Average fat; fat counts vary widely among brands and recipes.

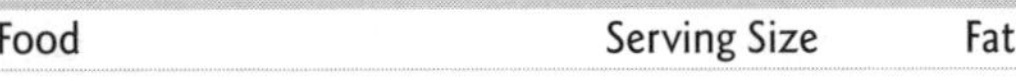

Food	Serving Size	Fat
Muffins and Quick Breads *(continued)*		
blueberry muffin	2½" × 2¼"	3.75
toaster muffin	1.4 oz	3.75
Boston brown bread	1 slice	.75
bran muffin	2 oz	5
carrot bread	2 oz slice	10
corn		
bread	2½" × 1½" piece	5
muffin	2½" × 2¼" piece	5
toaster muffin	1.4 oz	5.75
date nut bread	1 oz slice	2
hush puppy	1 piece	3
oat bran muffin	2 oz	4.25
scone	2 oz	7.5
shortcake	2 oz	9
Pizza*		
crust	1 lb; 12" diam	24

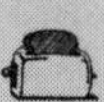

*Average fat; fat counts vary widely among brands, restaurants, and recipes.

Food	Serving Size	Fat
Pizza *(continued)*		
cheese only	slice	7
	12" pie	56
pepperoni	slice	9
	12" pie	72
sausage	slice	11
	12" pie	88
mushroom	slice	5
	12" pie	40
onion	slice	6
	12" pie	48
focaccia	2 oz	5
Pancakes, Waffles, French Toast*		
pancake		
blueberry	4" cake	3.5
buckwheat	4" cake	2.25
buttermilk	4" cake	3.5
plain	4" cake	3.5
whole wheat	4" cake	3

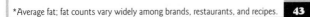

*Average fat; fat counts vary widely among brands, restaurants, and recipes.

Food	Serving Size	Fat
Pancakes, Waffles, French Toast *(continued)*		
waffles		
home made or mix	7" diam	10.5
frozen, toaster style	4" diam	2.75
french toast		
home recipe	slice	7
frozen	slice	3.5
Taco and Tortilla Shells*		
burrito	12" diam	5
corn tortilla	7" diam	.5
flour tortilla	8" diam	2.5
taco shell	5" diam	3
Wraps		
egg roll, raw	1 oz	0
lahvash	1 oz	0
wonton, raw	7" square	tr

*Average fat; fat counts vary widely among brands.

Food	Serving Size	Fat
Cereals*		
Alpha Bits	1 cup	1
Apple Jacks	1 cup	tr
bran		
all bran	½ cup	1
extra fiber	½ cup	.5
raisin nut	½ cup	3
flakes	1 oz	.5
flakes, with raisins	1 cup	1.5
buds	1 oz	.75
Cap'n Crunch	1 oz	1.5
Cheerios		
regular	1 cup	2
apple cinnamon	¾ cup	2
honey nut	1 cup	1.5
multi-grain	1 cup	1
Chex		
corn	1 oz	2
multi-bran	2 oz	2
rice	1 oz	0
wheat	¾ cup	1
Cocoa Crispies	¾ cup	.75
Cocoa Puffs	1 cup	1

*Average fat; fat counts vary widely among brands.

Food	Serving Size	Fat
Cereals *(continued)*		
corn		
flakes	1 cup	.25
frosted flakes	¾ cup	2
pops	1 cup	.25
Count Chocula	1 cup	1
cream of rice, cooked	¾ cup	.25
cream of wheat, cooked	¾ cup	.5
Crispix	1 cup	.25
Froot Loops	1 cup	1
Fruit and Fibre	1 cup	3
graham		
cinnamon	¾ cup	1
golden	¾ cup	1
granola	1 oz	7
Grape Nuts	½ cup	1
flakes	¾ cup	1
kasha, puffed	1 cup	.5
Kix	1⅓ cup	.5
Life	¾ cup	1.25

Food	Serving Size	Fat
Cereals *(continued)*		
muesli		
regular	½ cup	3
no sugar added	½ cup	3
multigrain flakes	¾ cup	1
oat bran	¾ cup	1.25
oatmeal (also see *Grains: oats*)		
regular, rolled, cooked	1 cup	2.25
instant, cooked	1 packet	1.75
flavored	1 packet	2
rice		
crisps	1¼ cup	2
frosted	1 cup	.25
puffed	1 cup	tr
Special K	1 cup	.25
Total	¾ cup	1
Trix	1 cup	1.5
wheat		
shredded	1 oz	.5
mini	1 cup	.5
mini, sugar coated	1 cup	1
flakes	1 cup	tr
sugar coated	¾ cup	.25
puffed	1 cup	.25

Food	Serving Size	Fat
Cereals *(continued)*		
Wheatena, cooked	3/4 cup	1
Wheaties	1 cup	1
Grains		
barley		
uncooked	1/4 cup	1
cooked	1 cup	.75
buckwheat groats, roasted (kasha)		
uncooked	1 cup	3.75
cooked	1 cup	1.25
bulgur (see *wheat, cracked*)		
corn kernels (see *Snack Foods: popcorn*)		
corn meal	1 cup	4.5
couscous		
uncooked	1 cup	tr
cooked	1 cup	tr
farina		
uncooked	1 oz	tr
cooked	1 cup	.25
flours (see *Sweets and Desserts: Baking Ingredients*)		

Food	Serving Size	Fat
Grains *(continued)*		
grits (corn)		
uncooked	¼ cup	0
cooked	1 cup	.5
kasha (see *buckwheat groats*)		
matzo meal	1 cup	2
millet		
uncooked	1 oz	1.25
cooked	1 cup	2.5
oat bran		
uncooked	½ cup	3.25
cooked	½ cup	1
oatmeal (see *Cereals*)		
oats		
rolled, uncooked	½ cup	3
rolled, cooked	1 cup	2.25
steel cut, uncooked	⅓ cup	4.5
polenta (see *cornmeal*)		
quinoa, uncooked	½ cup	5
rye		
whole grain	½ cup	2
flakes	⅓ cup	.5
flour (see *Sweets and Desserts: Baking Ingredients*)		

Food	Serving Size	Fat
Grains *(continued)*		
tabbouleh (see *wheat, cracked*)		
tapioca, dry	⅓ cup	0
wheat		
berries, kernels	1 cup	1.25
bran	½ cup	1.25
cracked (bulgur, tabbouleh)		
uncooked	½ cup	1
cooked	1 cup	.5
germ	¼ cup	3
Rice*		
arborio (see *white, short grain*)		
basmati (see *white, long grain*)		
brown		
uncooked	1 cup	5
cooked	1 cup	1.5
jasmine (see *white, long grain*)		
sushi (see *white, short grain*)		

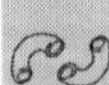

*For rice dishes, see *Soups, Stews, Casseroles, and Other Combination Foods.*

Food	Serving Size	Fat
Rice *(continued)*		
white		
short grain		
uncooked	1 cup	1
cooked	1 cup	.5
long grain		
uncooked	1 cup	1
cooked	1 cup	.5
instant		
uncooked	½ cup	0
cooked	½ cup	0
wild		
uncooked	1 cup	13
cooked	1 cup	.5
Pasta*		
dry pasta (all shapes)		
dry	2 oz	1.25
cooked	1 cup	1
fresh pasta		
uncooked	4 oz	2.5
cooked	1 cup	1
filled pasta		
ravioli		
meat	3 oz; 1 cup	9
cheese	3 oz; 1 cup	9

*For pasta dishes, see *Soups, Stews, Casseroles, and Other Combination Foods*.

Food	Serving Size	Fat
Pasta *(continued)*		
filled pasta *(continued)*		
tortellini, cheese	3 oz; ¾ cup	6
macaroni		
dry	2 oz	1.25
cooked	1 cup	11
noodles		
chow mein	1 cup	3.75
egg noodles		
dry	2 oz	2.5
cooked	1 cup	2.5
egg noodles, yolk free		
dry	2 oz	1
cooked	1 cup	1
rice (cellophane), dry	1 oz	0
soba (buckwheat)		
dry	1 oz	.5
cooked	1 cup	.5

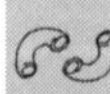

Food	Serving Size	Fat
Milk		
whole (3.5% fat)	8 oz	8
light, reduced fat (2% fat)	8 oz	4.75
low fat (1% fat)	8 oz	2.5
skim, fat free (0% fat)	8 oz	.5
buttermilk, low fat (1% fat)	8 oz	2.25
chocolate milk		
whole (3.5% fat)	8 oz	8.5
reduced fat (2% fat)	8 oz	5
low fat (1%)	8 oz	2.5
cocoa, chocolate drinks, and drink mixes (see *Beverages*)		
condensed, sweetened		
regular	2 tbsp	3.5
	1 cup	26.5
low fat	2 tbsp	1.5
	1 cup	12
fat free	2 tbsp	0
	1 cup	0
dry		
whole, powder	1 cup	34
	¼ cup	8.5
skim, nonfat, powder	1 cup	1
	¼ cup	tr
reconstituted	1 cup	tr

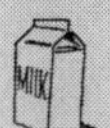

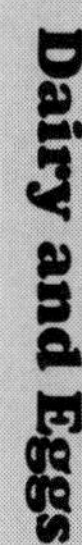

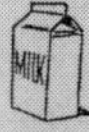

Food	Serving Size	Fat
Milk *(continued)*		
evaporated		
whole	1 cup	19
	2 tbsp	2.5
low fat (1% fat)	1 cup	4
	2 tbsp	.5
skim, fat free (0% fat)	1 cup	1
	2 tbsp	tr
rice (see *Diet and Health Foods: Milk Substitutes*)		
soy (see *Diet and Health Foods: Milk Substitutes*)		
Cream		
crème fraîche	2 tbsp	11
half and half	1 cup	28
	1 oz	3.5
heavy	1 cup	88
	2 tbsp	11
ice cream (see *Sweets and Desserts*)		
light	1 cup	46
	2 tbsp	6
mascarpone	1 oz	13

Food	Serving Size	Fat
Cream *(continued)*		
sour		
whole	1 cup	48
	1 tbsp	2.5
reduced fat	1 cup	29
	1 tbsp	2
fat free	1 cup	tr
	1 tbsp	tr
imitation	1 cup	45
	1 tbsp	5.5
sour cream dips (see *Snack Foods*)		
whipped*		
fresh	1 cup	44
	1 tbsp	3
pressurized	1 cup	13
	1 tbsp	1
nondairy topping		
regular, extra creamy	2 tbsp	2
light	2 tbsp	1
fat free	2 tbsp	0
powdered	2½ g	.5
mix	2 tbsp	.5
reconstituted with 2% milk	1 cup	10

*Average fat; fat counts vary widely among brands.

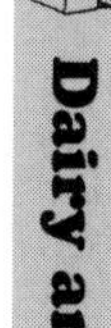

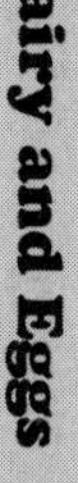

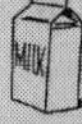

Food	Serving Size	Fat
Nondairy creamers*		
liquid		
regular	1 tbsp	1.5
flavored	1 tbsp	2
fat free	1 tbsp	0
flavored	1 tbsp	0
powdered	1 tsp	1
Shakes		
nutritional (see *Diet and Health Foods)*		
smoothies (see *Beverages)*		
thick, milk, malted (see *Sweets and Desserts)*		
Yogurt*		
plain		
whole	8 oz container	7
low fat	8 oz container	3.5
nonfat	8 oz container	.5
flavored (coffee, vanilla)		
low fat	8 oz container	2.75
nonfat	8 oz container	0
with fruit		
low fat	8 oz container	3
nonfat	8 oz container	0

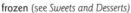

frozen (see *Sweets and Desserts)*

*Average fat; fat counts vary widely among brands.

Food	Serving Size	Fat
Cheese*		
American		
regular	1 oz	9
	slice; 21 g	5
light, reduced fat	slice; 21 g	3
fat free	slice; 21 g	0
lactose free (nondairy)	slice; 19 g	0
Asiago	1 oz	8
blue (including Roquefort, Stilton, Gorgonzola, Danish)	1 oz	8
crumbled	1 cup	35
Boursin	1 oz	13
light	1 oz	3
brick	1 oz	8.5
Brie	1 oz	8
Camembert	1 oz	7
caraway	1 oz	8
Cheddar		
regular	1 oz	9.5
shredded	1 cup	38
low fat	1 oz	2
shredded	1 cup	8

*Average fat; fat counts vary widely among brands.

Food	Serving Size	Fat
Cheese *(continued)*		
cheese dip (see *Snack Foods)*		
cheese food		
(prepared cheese product, Velveeta)	1 oz	6
cheese sauce (see *Extras: Sauces*)		
cheese spread (American)	1 oz	6
light	1 oz	3
chèvre (see *goat cheese)*		
colby		
regular	1 oz	9
shredded	1 cup	36
low fat	1 oz	2
shredded	1 cup	8
cottage cheese		
plain, creamed (4% fat)	4 oz	5
plain, reduced fat (2% fat)	4 oz	2
plain, low fat (1% fat)	4 oz	1
plain, nonfat (0% fat)	4 oz	.5
with fruit, creamed (4% fat)	4 oz	2
with fruit, low fat (1% fat)	4 oz	1
with fruit, nonfat (0% fat)	4 oz	0
cream cheese		
regular	1 oz	10
light, Neufchâtel	1 oz	6.5
fat free	1 oz	.5

Food	Serving Size	Fat
Cheese *(continued)*		
cream cheese *(continued)*		
whipped	1 tbsp	3.5
flavored	1 tbsp	3
Edam	1 oz	8
farmer	1 oz	2.5
feta	1 oz	6
crumbled	1 cup	32
fondue	½ cup	14.5
fontina	1 oz	9
gjetost	1 oz	8
goat		
hard	1 oz	10
soft	1 oz	6.8
Gouda	1 oz	8
Gruyère (see *Swiss)*		
Havarti	1 oz	11
jack	1 oz	8.5
Jarlsberg *(see Swiss)*		

Food	Serving Size	Fat
Cheese *(continued)*		
Limburger	1 oz	8
mozzarella		
whole milk	1 oz	6
shredded	1 cup	24
part skim	1 oz	4.5
shredded	1 oz	18
Muenster	1 oz	8.5
Neufchâtel (see *cream cheese)*		
Parmesan, grated	1 oz	8.5
	1 cup	30
Port Salut	1 oz	8
provolone	1 oz	7.5
ricotta		
whole milk	1 cup	32
part skim	1 cup	20
Romano	1 oz	7.5
string	1 oz	6
Swiss (Gruyère, Jarlsberg)	1 oz	8

Food	Serving Size	Fat
Cheese *(continued)*		
Tilsit	1 oz	7.5
wine Cheddar spread	1 oz	7
Eggs		
whole; raw, boiled, poached	large	5.5
	extra large	6
	jumbo	6.5
white	from 1 large egg	0
yolk	from 1 large egg	5
powdered		
whole	1 cup	35
	1 tbsp	2
white	1 cup	tr
	1 tbsp	0
yolk	1 cup	38
	1 tbsp	2
deviled	1 whole	13
fried	1 large egg	7
omelet	2 large eggs	14
scrambled	1 large egg	7.5

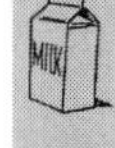

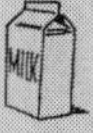

Food	Serving Size	Fat
Eggs *(continued)*		
egg nog (see *Beverages*)		
egg substitutes		
frozen	1 cup	27
liquid	1 cup	8.5
powder	.7 oz	2.5

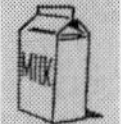

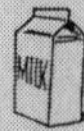

Food	Serving Size	Fat
Diet Foods: Nutritional Shakes*		
Boost	8 oz	4
Carnation Instant Breakfast		
regular, powder	1 envelope	1
no sugar added, powder	1 envelope	1
ready to drink	10 oz	3
Ensure		
regular	8 oz	8.75
plus	8 oz	12.5
Met-Rx, powder	2½ oz	2
Nutrament	1 can	3
Sweet Success, powder	1 scoop	.75
Ultra Slim-Fast		
powder	1.2 oz	1
can	11 oz	3
Diet Foods: Diet Bars*		
Boost	1 bar	6
Carnation Breakfast	1.27 oz bar	6
Figurine	2 bars	11

*For low-fat, reduced-fat, light, and sugar-free foods, see main categories for each.

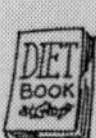

Food	Serving Size	Fat
Diet Foods: Diet Bars *(continued)*		
Met-RX	3½ oz bar	3
Nature Valley, low fat	1 oz bar	2
Nutrigrain	1⅓ oz bar	0
Sweet Rewards, fat free	1⅓ oz bar	2.75
Sweet Success	1 bar	3.25
Ultra Slim-Fast	1 oz bar	4
Other Diet Foods		
diet soft drinks (see *Beverages*)		
sugar free candy (see *Snack Foods*)		
Health Foods		
brewer's yeast	1 oz	.25
lecithin granules	1 tbsp	5
meat and poultry substitutes (see *Meats and Poultry*)		
milk substitutes*		
rice milk	1 cup	3
soy milk		
regular	1 cup	5

*Average fat; fat counts vary widely among brands.

Food	Serving Size	Fat
Health Foods *(continued)*		
milk substitutes *(continued)*		
soy milk *(continued)*		
unsweetened	1 cup	4.5
light	1 cup	2
low fat	1 cup	2
nonfat	1 cup	0
seaweed		
kelp, raw	3½ oz	.5
laver, raw	3½ oz	.25
spirulina, raw	3½ oz	.5
soy grits	1 tbsp	1.5
tempeh	½ cup	6.5
tofu		
cake	1 oz	1.5
cream (sour cream substitute)	2 tbsp	5
frozen dessert (see *Sweets and Desserts)*		
spread (cream cheese substitute)	1 oz	8

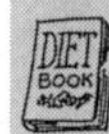

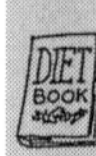

Food	Serving Size	Fat
Dressings*		
bleu cheese		
regular	1 tbsp	8
	1 cup	128
reduced fat	1 tbsp	3.25
	1 cup	52
made from mix	1 tbsp	8
	1 cup	128
buttermilk		
ranch style	1 tbsp	8
	1 cup	128
from mix	1 tbsp	6
	1 cup	96
caesar		
regular	1 tbsp	7
	1 cup	112
reduced calorie	1 tbsp	2.5
	1 cup	40
made from mix	1 tbsp	8
	1 cup	128
catalina		
regular	1 tbsp	6.5
	1 cup	104
fat free	1 tbsp	2
	1 cup	32

*Average fat; fat counts vary widely among brands and recipes.

Food	Serving Size	Fas
Dressings *(continued)*		
cole slaw	1 tbsp	6
	1 cup	96
French (creamy)		
regular	1 tbsp	6
	1 cup	96
reduced calorie	1 tbsp	1.5
	1 cup	24
fat free	1 tbsp	tr
	1 cup	15
green goddess	1 tbsp	6.5
	1 cup	104
herb	1 tbsp	6
	1 cup	96
honey mustard		
regular or made from mix	1 tbsp	7.5
	1 cup	120
fat free	1 tbsp	0
	1 cup	tr
made from mix	1 tbsp	0
	1 cup	tr
Italian		
regular and made from mix	1 tbsp	7
	1 cup	112
reduced fat	1 tbsp	1.5
	1 cup	24

Food	Serving Size	Fat
Dressings *(continued)*		
mayonnaise		
regular	1 tbsp	11
	1 cup	174.5
reduced fat, light	1 tbsp	5
	1 cup	80
fat free	1 tbsp	.5
	1 cup	8
Miracle Whip		
regular	1 tbsp	7
	1 cup	112
light	1 tbsp	3
	1 cup	48
fat free	1 tbsp	0
	1 cup	tr
ranch		
regular	1 tbsp	9
	1 cup	144
made from mix	1 tbsp	6
	1 cup	96
fat free	1 tbsp	0
	1 cup	tr
reduced calorie, made from mix	1 tbsp	2.25
	1 cup	36
Russian		
regular	1 tbsp	7.5
	1 cup	120
reduced fat	1 tbsp	.5
	1 cup	9.5

Food	Serving Size	Fat
Dressings *(continued)*		
thousand island		
regular	1 tbsp	5.75
	1 cup	90
reduced fat	1 tbsp	1.5
	1 cup	24
vinaigrette, oil and vinegar		
home recipe	1 tbsp	8
	1 cup	128
regular	1 tbsp	5.5
	1 cup	88
fat free	1 tbsp	0
	1 cup	tr
vinegar (see *Condiments*)		
Gravy*		
au jus		
canned	2 tbsp	tr
	1 cup	.5
made from mix	2 tbsp	tr
	1 cup	1
beef, canned	2 tbsp	.5
	1 cup	4

*Average fat; fat counts vary widely among brands and recipes.

Food	Serving Size	Fat
Gravy *(continued)*		
brown		
canned	2 tbsp	1
	1 cup	9
made from mix	2 tbsp	.25
	1 cup	2
chicken		
canned	2 tbsp	1.5
	1 cup	12.5
made from mix	2 tbsp	.5
	1 cup	2.25
cream	2 tbsp	1
	1 cup	7
mushroom		
canned	2 tbsp	.5
	1 cup	3
made from mix	2 tbsp	tr
	1 cup	1
onion		
canned	2 tbsp	.5
	1 cup	3.25
made from mix	2 tbsp	tr
	1 cup	.75
pork		
canned	2 tbsp	1
	1 cup	8

Food	Serving Size	Fat
Gravy *(continued)*		
pork *(continued)*		
made from mix	2 tbsp	.25
	1 cup	2
turkey		
canned	2 tbsp	.5
	1 cup	3.5
made from mix	2 tbsp	.25
	1 cup	2
Sauces*		
Alfredo	2 tbsp	8
	1 cup	64
black bean	1 tbsp	1
brown	2 tbsp	3.5
	1 cup	26.5
cheese	2 tbsp	4.5
	1 cup	36
clam		
red	2 tbsp	.25
	1 cup	2
white	2 tbsp	2.5
	1 cup	20

*Average calories; calorie counts vary widely among brands and recipes.

Food	Serving Size	Fat
Sauces *(continued)*		
curry	2 tbsp	1.25
	1 cup	10
hollandaise	2 tbsp	9
	1 cup	36
mole poblano	2 tbsp	3.5
	1 cup	26.5
nacho cheese	2 tbsp	4
	1 cup	32
pesto	2 tbsp	6.5
	1 cup	52.5
pizza	2 tbsp	tr
	1 cup	2
sloppy joe	¼ cup	.75
	1 cup	3
teriyaki	2 tbsp	0
	1 cup	0
tomato		
homemade	2 tbsp	.2
	1 cup	1.5
canned, jarred	2 tbsp	.5
	1 cup	5

Food	Serving Size	Fat
Sauces *(continued)*		
white		
thin	2 tbsp	2
	1 cup	17
medium	2 tbsp	3.25
	1 cup	26.5
thick	2 tbsp	4.5
	1 cup	34.5
Condiments*		
barbecue sauce	1 tbsp	.5
	1 cup	4.5
capers	1 tbsp	0
catsup (see *ketchup*)		
chili sauce	2 tbsp	tr
	1 cup	1
chutney	2 tbsp	0
cocktail sauce (ketchup based)	2 tbsp	.25
	1 cup	2
hoisin sauce	½ cup	tr
horseradish	1 tbsp	0

*Average calories; calorie counts vary widely among brands and recipes.

Food	Serving Size	Fat
Condiments *(continued)*		
ketchup	1 tbsp	tr
mustard		
American style	1 tsp	tr
French style	1 tsp	0
honey	1 tsp	0
relish		
sweet pickle	1 tbsp	.5
hot dog	1 tbsp	tr
remoulade	2 tbsp	11
salsa	2 tbsp	tr
soy sauce	1 tbsp	0
steak sauce	1 tbsp	0
sweet and sour	2 tbsp	0
Tabasco	1 tsp	0
taco	1 tbsp	0
tartar sauce		
regular	2 tbsp	10
nonfat	2 tbsp	0

Food	Serving Size	Fat
Condiments *(continued)*		
vinegar		
balsamic, red wine, flavored, herb	1 tbsp	0
cider, white	1 tbsp	0
Worcestershire sauce	1 tsp	0
Flavorings		
Accent	1 tsp	0
adobo	1 tsp	0
bitters	½ tsp	0
bouillon cubes	1 cube	0
broth powder	1 tsp	0
butter flavoring	1 tsp	0
extracts		
almond	1 tsp	0
orange	1 tsp	0
mint	1 tsp	0
vanilla	1 tsp	0
miso	1 tbsp	1
	1 cup	17

Food	Serving Size	Fat
Herbs and Spices		
allspice, ground	1 tsp	2.5
anise seed	1 tsp	2.5
basil		
fresh	2 tbsp	0
dried	1 tsp	0
bay leaf	1 leaf	tr
caraway seed	1 tsp	.25
celery seed	1 tsp	.5
chervil, dried	1 tsp	0
chili powder	1 tsp	.5
Chinese parsley (see *coriander*)		
chives		
fresh, chopped	1 tbsp	0
dried, freeze dried	¼ tsp	0
cilantro (see *coriander*)		
cinnamon, ground	1 tsp	tr
cloves, ground	1 tsp	.5

Food	Serving Size	Fat
Herbs and Spices *(continued)*		
coriander (cilantro, Chinese parsley)		
fresh leaf	¼ cup	0
dried leaf	1 tsp	0
seed	1 tsp	.5
cumin		
ground	1 tsp	tr
seed	1 tsp	.5
curry powder	1 tsp	.5
dill		
seed	1 tsp	.5
weed, fresh	1 cup	0
weed, dried	1 tsp	tr
fennel seed	1 tsp	.5
garlic (see *Vegetables*)		
garlic powder	1 tsp	0
ginger		
fresh root	¼ cup	tr
ground	1 tsp	tr
mace	1 tsp	.5
marjoram, dried	1 tsp	tr

Food	Serving Size	Fat
Herbs and Spices *(continued)*		
mustard		
powder	1 tsp	1
seed	1 tsp	1
nutmeg, ground	1 tsp	.5
onion powder	1 tsp	0
oregano, dried	1 tsp	tr
paprika	1 tsp	.5
parsley		
fresh	½ cup	tr
dried	1 tsp	0
pepper, ground black, red, white	1 tsp	.25
poppy seed	1 tsp	1.25
poultry seasoning	1 tsp	.25
rosemary, dried	1 tsp	.25
saffron	1 tsp	tr
sage, dried, rubbed	1 tsp	tr
salt and **salt substitutes**	1 tsp	0
savory, ground	1 tsp	tr

Food	Serving Size	Fat
Herbs and Spices *(continued)*		
shallots (see *Vegetables*)		
tarragon, dried	1 tsp	tr
thyme		
fresh	1 tsp	0
dried	1 tsp	tr
turmeric, ground	1 tsp	.25

Food	Serving Size	Fat
Fats		
butter		
salted or unsalted	1 tbsp	12
	1 stick; ¼ lb; ½ cup	95
whipped	1 tbsp	7.5
	1 cup	122.5
light (margarine/butter blend)	1 tbsp	11.5
	1 stick; ¼ lb; ½ cup	92
margarine		
regular	1 tbsp	11.5
	1 stick; ¼ lb; ½ cup	92
soft (tub)	1 tbsp	11.5
	1 cup	182.5
liquid	1 tbsp	6
	1 cup	90
substitutes		
Benecol	1 tbsp	9
Brummel & Brown	1 tbsp	5
I Can't Believe It's Not Butter	1 tbsp	10
light	1 tbsp	6
Olivio	1 tbsp	8
Smart Balance	1 tbsp	9
Smartbeat	1 tbsp	2
Take Control	1 tbsp	6
light	1 tbsp	4.5

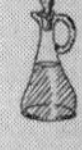

Food	Serving Size	Fat
Fats *(continued)*		
chicken fat	1 tbsp	13
	1 cup	205
duck fat *(see chicken fat)*		
goose fat *(see chicken fat)*		
lard	1 tbsp	13
	1 cup	205
salt pork	1 oz	22.75
shortening (solid)		
vegetable oil	1 tbsp	13
	1 cup	205
vegetable oil/lard blend	1 tbsp	13
	1 cup	205
suet (beef)	1 oz	26.5
tallow (beef, mutton)	1 tbsp	13
	1 cup	205
turkey fat *(see chicken fat)*		
Oils		
canola (rapeseed)	1 tbsp	14
	1 cup	218

Food	Serving Size	Fat
Oils *(continued)*		
cocoa butter	1 tbsp	13.5
	1 cup	218
coconut	1 tbsp	13.5
	1 cup	218
cod liver *(see fish oil)*		
corn	1 tbsp	13.5
	1 cup	218
cottonseed	1 tbsp	13.5
	1 cup	218
fish oil (cod liver, herring, menhaden, salmon)	1 tbsp	14
grapeseed	1 tbsp	13.5
	1 cup	218
olive	1 tbsp	13.5
	1 cup	216
nut (almond, apricot kernel, hazelnut, walnut)	1 tbsp	14
	1 cup	224
palm	1 tbsp	13.5
	1 cup	216

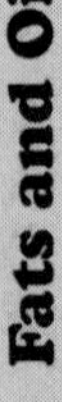

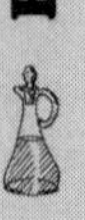

Food	Serving Size	Fat
Oils *(continued)*		
peanut	1 tbsp	13.5
	1 cup	216
safflower	1 tbsp	13.5
	1 cup	218
sesame	1 tbsp	13.5
	1 cup	218
soybean	1 tbsp	13.5
	1 cup	218
spray	1 spray	.25
sunflower	1 tbsp	13.5
	1 cup	218
vegetable (blended)	1 tbsp	13.5
	1 cup	218
wheat germ	1 tbsp	13.5
	1 cup	218

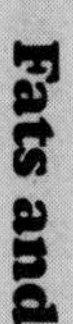

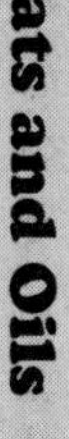

Food	Serving Size	Fat
Note: Edible portions only; no bones or shells.		
abalone		
raw	3 oz	.5
fried	3 oz	6
anchovy		
raw, free	3 oz	4
canned, in oil	5 filets	2
paste	1 tsp	1
bass		
black		
raw	4 oz	1.5
steamed, poached, broiled, grilled, baked, microwaved	3½ oz	1.5
sautéed	3½ oz	8.5
Chilean sea bass (see *grouper*)		
striped		
raw	4 oz	2.5
steamed, poached, broiled, grilled, baked, microwaved	3½ oz	2.5
sautéed	3½ oz	9.5
blackfish (see *tautog*)		
bluefish		
raw	4 oz	4.75
steamed, poached, broiled, grilled, baked, microwaved	3½ oz	4.75

Food	Serving Size	Fat
butterfish		
raw	4 oz	9
sautéed	3½ oz	16
calamari (squid)		
raw	4 oz	1.5
grilled	3½ oz	1.5
fried	3 oz	6.5
carp		
raw	4 oz	6.5
poached	3½ oz	6.5
fried, sautéed	3½ oz	13.5
catfish		
raw	4 oz	8.5
broiled	3½ oz	8
fried, breaded	4 oz	15
caviar, black or red	1 tbsp	3
clams		
raw	3 oz	.75
steamed	3 oz	1.75
fried, breaded	4 oz	9.5
canned, drained	3 oz	1.75
clam juice	1 cup	0
cod		
raw	4 oz	.5
steamed, poached, broiled,		

Food	Serving Size	Fat
cod *(continued)*		
baked, microwaved	3½ oz	.75
sautéed	3½ oz	7.75
salt (dried)	3 oz	2
crab		
Alaska king, steamed or boiled	3 oz	1.25
blue, steamed or boiled	3 oz	1.5
Dungeness, steamed or boiled	3 oz	1
legs, imitation (see *surimi*)		
crayfish, boiled	3 oz	1
croaker		
raw	4 oz	3.5
fried, breaded	4 oz	12.5
dolphin fish (see *mahi-mahi*)		
dover sole (see *flounder*)		
eel		
raw	4 oz	13.25
grilled, poached, microwaved	3½ oz	15
smoked	3 oz	24
finnan haddie (see *haddock, smoked*)		
fish filets, frozen		
battered	4 oz	17
lightly battered	3⅓ oz	10.5

Food	Serving Size	Fat
fish sticks, frozen	3 oz	10.25
flounder (sole)		
raw	4 oz	1.25
grilled, poached, microwaved	3½ oz	1.25
fried, breaded	4 oz	13
gefilte fish		
regular	2 oz	2
with jelled broth	2 oz	2
sweet	2 oz	2
with jelled broth	2 oz	2
grouper (rock cod, Chilean sea bass)		
raw	4 oz	1.25
steamed, poached, broiled, grilled, baked, microwaved	3½ oz	1.25
sautéed	3½ oz	8.25
fried, breaded	3½ oz	13
haddock		
raw	4 oz	1
steamed, poached, broiled, baked, grilled, microwaved	3½ oz	1
sautéed	3½ oz	8
smoked (finnan haddie)	3 oz	1

hake (see *whiting*)

Food	Serving Size	Fat
halibut		
raw	4 oz	3
steamed, poached, broiled, grilled, baked, microwaved	3½ oz	2
sautéed	3½ oz	9
herring		
raw	4 oz	7.75
grilled, broiled	3½ oz	11.5
pickled	1 oz	4
pickled, in sour cream	1 oz	5
smoked (kippered)	2 oz	7
canned	2 oz	7
with tomato sauce	2 oz	6
kingfish (see *mackerel*)		
ling		
raw	4 oz	.5
steamed, poached, broiled, baked, microwaved	3½ oz	.75
sautéed	3½ oz	7.75
fried, breaded	4 oz	17
lobster		
raw	4 oz	1
boiled, steamed, broiled, baked	3 oz	.5
lox (see *salmon, smoked*)		

Food	Serving Size	Fat
mackerel		
raw	4 oz	7
grilled, broiled	3½ oz	6
mahi-mahi (dolphin fish)		
raw	4 oz	.75
steamed, poached, broiled, baked, grilled, microwaved	3½ oz	1
sautéed	3½ oz	8
mako (see *shark*)		
monkfish (lotte)		
raw	4 oz	1.75
steamed, poached, broiled, baked, grilled, microwaved	3½ oz	2
sautéed	3½ oz	9
mullet		
raw	4 oz	1.75
sautéed	3½ oz	10
fried, breaded	4 oz	12
mussels		
raw	4 oz	2.5
steamed	4 oz	5
Nova Scotia (see *salmon, smoked)*		
octopus		
raw	4 oz	1
boiled	3½ oz	2

Food	Serving Size	Fat
orange roughy		
raw	4 oz	.75
steamed, poached, broiled, baked, microwaved	3½ oz	1
sautéed	3½ oz	8
oysters		
raw	3 oz; 6 medium	2
fried, breaded	3 oz; 6 medium	10.75
Rockefeller	6	26
perch		
raw	4 oz	1
steamed, poached, broiled, baked, microwaved	3½ oz	1
sautéed	3½ oz	9
fried, breaded	4 oz	13
pike (pickerel)		
raw	4 oz	1
sautéed	3½ oz	8
fried, breaded	4 oz	12
plaice (see *flounder*)		
pollack		
raw	4 oz	1
steamed, poached, broiled, baked, microwaved	3½ oz	1.25
sautéed	3½ oz	9

Food	Serving Size	Fat
pompano		
raw	4 oz	10
grilled, poached, microwaved	3½ oz	12
sautéed	3½ oz	20
porgy		
raw	4 oz	4
poached, broiled, microwaved	3½ oz	4
sautéed	3½ oz	11
fried, breaded	4 oz	16
rockfish (see *bass, striped*)		
sable, smoked	3 oz	17
salmon (pink)		
raw	4 oz	4
steamed, poached, broiled, baked, grilled, microwaved	3½ oz	4.5
sautéed	3½ oz	12
canned	3 oz	6
salmon (red)		
raw	4 oz	10
steamed, poached, broiled, baked, grilled, microwaved	3½ oz	12
sautéed	3½ oz	20
canned	3 oz	9
smoked (lox, nova scotia, scotch)	3 oz	3.75

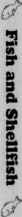

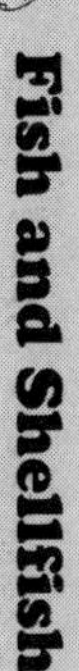

Food	Serving Size	Fat
scallops		
raw	3 oz	.75
poached, steamed, baked, grilled, broiled, microwaved	3 oz	1
sautéed	3 oz	9
fried, breaded	3 oz	10
scrod (see *haddock*)		
scup (see *porgy*)		
shad		
raw	4 oz	15.5
broiled	3½ oz	17
sautéed	3½ oz	22
roe		
raw	3 oz	5.5
sautéed	3 oz	13
shark (mako)		
raw	4 oz	6
grilled, broiled, poached	3½ oz	6
sautéed	3½ oz	14
shrimp		
raw	3 oz; 12 large	1.5
poached, boiled, steamed, baked, grilled, broiled, microwaved	3 oz; 15 large	1
sautéed	3 oz; 12 large	8.5
fried, breaded	3 oz; 11 large	10.5

Food	Serving Size	Fat
skate (ray)		
raw	4 oz	.75
poached	3½ oz	.75
sautéed	3½ oz	8
smelt		
raw	4 oz	3
broiled	3½ oz	2.75
sautéed	3½ oz	11
fried, breaded	4 oz	14
snapper		
raw	4 oz	1.5
poached, boiled, steamed, baked, microwaved, grilled, broiled	3½ oz	1.75
sautéed	3½ oz	9
fried, breaded	4 oz	11
sole *(see flounder)*		
squid *(see calamari)*		
sturgeon		
raw	4 oz	4.5
grilled, baked, poached, microwaved	3½ oz	4.5
smoked	3 oz	3.75
surimi (imitation crab legs)	3 oz	1
swordfish		
raw	4 oz	4.5

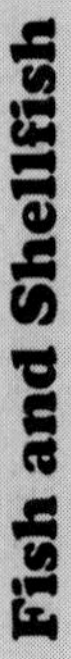

Food	Serving Size	Fat
swordfish *(continued)*		
grilled, broiled, poached, baked, microwaved	3½ oz	5
sautéed	3½ oz	12
tautog (blackfish)		
raw	4 oz	1.25
grilled, broiled, poached, baked, microwaved	3½ oz	2
sautéed	3½ oz	9
tilefish		
raw	4 oz	2.5
poached, boiled, steamed, baked, broiled, microwaved	3½ oz	4.5
sautéed	3½ oz	12
trout		
brook, rainbow		
raw	4 oz	6
poached, steamed, microwaved, baked, broiled, grilled	3½ oz	7
sautéed	3½ oz	14
sea (weakfish)		
raw	4 oz	4
poached, steamed, microwaved, baked, broiled, grilled	3½ oz	4.5
sautéed	3½ oz	12
tuna		
albacore, bluefin		
raw	4 oz	6

Food	Serving Size	Fat
tuna *(continued)*		
albacore, bluefin *(continued)*		
grilled, broiled, baked, microwaved	3½ oz	5.75
sautéed	3½ oz	11
yellowfin, skipjack		
raw	4 oz	1
grilled, broiled, baked, microwaved	3½ oz	1
sautéed	3½ oz	6
canned		
light, in water	3 oz	.75
light, in oil, drained	3 oz	7
white, in water	3 oz	2.5
white, in oil, drained	3 oz	7
turbot		
raw	4 oz	3.25
poached, broiled, microwaved	3½ oz	3.75
sautéed	3½ oz	10
whitefish		
raw	4 oz	6.5
poached, broiled, microwaved	3½ oz	7.5
sautéed	3½ oz	15
smoked	3 oz	1
whiting (hake)		
raw	4 oz	1.5
poached, baked, microwaved	3½ oz	1.75
sautéed	3½ oz	9
fried, breaded	4 oz	15
yellowtail *(see pompano)*		

Food	Serving Size	Fat

Note: For fruit juices, see *Beverages*; for fruit pies and jams, jellies, preserves, and spreads, see *Sweets and Desserts*.

Food	Serving Size	Fat
apple		
whole, raw, with skin	small; 4 oz	.5
	medium; 5 oz	.5
	large; 7½ oz	.75
cooked, without skin	1 cup	.5
canned, sweetened, drained	1 cup	.5
caramel-covered	1 medium	1
dried	1 cup	.25

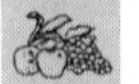

apple butter (see *Sweets and Desserts*)

apple pie (see *Sweets and Desserts*)

Fruits

Food	Serving Size	Fat
apple sauce		
regular	1 cup	.5
unsweetened, sugar free	1 cup	tr

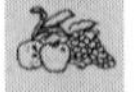

Food	Serving Size	Fat
apricot		
whole, raw	small; 1¼ oz	0
	medium; 2 oz	0
	large; 3 oz	0
candied	1 oz	0
canned		
in water	1 cup	.5
in light syrup	1 cup	tr
in heavy syrup	1 cup	.25
dried	1 cup	.75
	½ fruit	tr

Food	Serving Size	Fat
banana		
fresh		
small	4 oz, with skin	0
medium	5 oz, with skin	0
large	7 oz, with skin	0
mashed	1 cup	1
sliced	1 cup	.75
dried	1 cup	1.75
blackberries		
fresh	1 cup	.5
canned, in heavy syrup	1 cup	.25
frozen, unsweetened	1 cup	.5
blueberries		
fresh	1 cup	.5
	1 pint	1.5
canned, in heavy syrup	1 cup	.75
frozen		
unsweetened	1 cup	1
sweetened	1 cup	.25
boysenberries		
canned in heavy syrup	1 cup	.25
cantaloupe		
slice	2 oz, without skin	.25
pieces	1 cup	.5

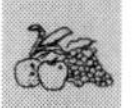

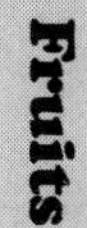

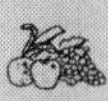

Food	Serving Size	Fat
casaba melon		
slice	6 oz, without skin	tr
pieces	1 cup	tr
cherries		
sour	1 cherry	tr
	1 lb	1
canned		
in light syrup	1 cup	.25
in heavy syrup	1 cup	.25
sweet	1 cherry	tr
	1 lb	1
canned		
in water	1 cup	.25
in light syrup	1 cup	.25
in heavy syrup	1 cup	.25
citrus peel		
fresh	1 tbsp	0
candied	1 oz	0
cranberries		
fresh, raw	1 cup	.25
jelly	1 cup	.5
whole fruit sauce	1 cup	0
dried	½ cup	0
currants		
fresh	1 cup	.25
dried	1 cup	.25

Food	Serving Size	Fat
dates		
fresh or dried	1 date	tr
pitted, chopped	1 cup	.75
figs		
fresh		
large	2½" diam	tr
medium	2¼" diam	tr
small	1½" diam	.25
canned		
in water	1 cup	tr
in light syrup	1 cup	tr
in heavy syrup	1 cup	tr
dried	1 fig	.25
fruit leather (see *Snack Foods: Candy*)		
fruit salad (fruit cocktail), canned		
in water	1 cup	tr
in light syrup	1 cup	tr
in heavy syrup	1 cup	tr
ginger (see *Extras: Herbs and Spices*)		
granadilla (see *passionfruit*)		
grapefruit	½ large; 4½" diam	tr
sections and juice	1 cup	.25
canned, in light syrup	1 cup	.25
grapes	1 grape	tr
	1 cup	1

Food	Serving Size	Fat
guava	1 cup	1
honeydew		
slice	3½ oz	tr
pieces	1 cup	tr
kiwi	1 fruit	.25
kumquat		
fresh	1 fruit	tr
canned, in heavy syrup	1 cup	.25
lemon	1 fruit	.25
lime	1 fruit	tr
mandarin		
fresh	1 large	tr
canned, in light syrup	1 cup	.25
mango		
fresh, flesh only	1 cup, slices	.5
dried	1 oz	0
nectarine	1 fruit; 2½" diam	.5
orange		
whole, fresh	small; 2½" diam	tr
	large; 3" diam	.25
sections	1 cup	.25
papaya	1 cup, cubes	.25

Food	Serving Size	Fat
passionfruit (granadilla)	1 fruit	tr
	1 cup, cubes	1.5
peach		
fresh, whole	large; 6½ oz	tr
	small; 4 oz	tr
canned		
in water	1 cup	tr
in light syrup	1 cup	tr
in heavy syrup	1 cup	.25
pear		
fresh, whole, all types	large; 8 oz	1
	small; 6 oz	.5
canned		
in water	1 cup	tr
in light syrup	1 cup	tr
in heavy syrup	1 cup	.25
dried	1 cup	1
	½ pear	tr
persimmon		
japanese, large	1 fruit	.25
american, small	1 fruit	tr
pineapple		
fresh, flesh only		
slice	⅛ pineapple	.25
diced	1 cup	.5
canned		
in water	1 cup	.25
	1 slice	tr

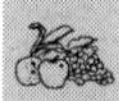
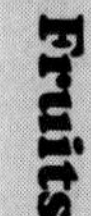

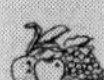

Food	Serving Size	Fat
pineapple *(continued)*		
canned *(continued)*		
in light syrup	1 cup	.25
	1 slice	tr
in heavy syrup	1 cup	.25
	1 slice	tr
dried	1 oz	0
plantain		
raw	1 cup	.5
cooked	1 cup	.25
plum		
damson	½ oz	0
all other types	2 oz	.5
canned, purple		
in water	1 cup	tr
in light syrup	1 cup	.25
in heavy syrup	1 cup	.25
pomegranate	1 fruit	.5
prickly pear	1 fruit	.5
prune		
dried, pitted	1 fruit	tr
	1 cup	1
stewed	1 cup	.5
canned, heavy syrup	1 cup	.5
quince	1 fruit	tr

Food	Serving Size	Fat
raisins	1 cup; 5 oz	.5
raspberries		
fresh, whole	10 berries	tr
	1 cup	1.5
	1 pint	1.75
frozen, sweetened	1 cup	.5
strawberries		
fresh	1 berry	tr
halves	1 cup	.5
purée, unsweetened	1 cup	.5
frozen		
whole, unsweetened	1 cup	.25
sliced, sweetened	1 cup	.25
tangerine	1 fruit	tr
watermelon		
slice	4 oz	tr
cubes	1 cup	.5

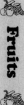

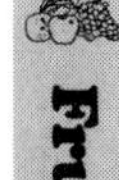
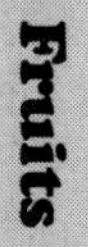
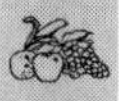

Food	Serving Size	Fat

Note: Edible portion, cooked as indicated, fat trim as indicated. Listings are for representative samples; values are approximate since degree of marbling (fat within meat) and trimming of surrounding fat, cooking temperature, and doneness vary.

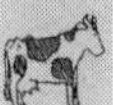

Meat: Beef

bologna (see *Luncheon and Deli Meats*)

brain (see *Organ Meats*)

Food	Serving Size	Fat
brisket		
whole, braised, lean and fat	3½ oz; ¼" fat trim	34.25
whole, braised, lean	3½ oz; 0" fat trim	10
chuck roast (pot roast)		
choice, braised, lean and fat	3½ oz; ¼" fat trim	26
choice, braised, lean	3½ oz; 0" fat trim	8.75
select, braised, lean and fat	3½ oz; ¼" fat trim	21.75
select, braised, lean	3½ oz; 0" fat trim	6.25
corned beef, cooked	3½ oz	19

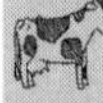

frankfurter (*see Luncheon and Deli Meats*)

Food	Serving Size	Fat
flank		
braised, lean and fat	3½ oz; 0" fat trim	16.5
braised, lean	3½ oz; 0" fat trim	13
broiled, lean and fat	3½ oz; 0" fat trim	12.5
broiled, lean	3½ oz; 0" fat trim	10

Food	Serving Size	Fat
Meat: Beef *(continued)*		
ground		
regular fat		
baked, medium-well	3 1/2 oz	21
broiled, medium-well	3 1/2 oz	20
pan fried, medium-well	3 1/2 oz	20.75
lean		
baked, medium-well	3 1/2 oz	21
broiled, medium-well	3 1/2 oz	20
pan fried, medium-well	3 1/2 oz	18.5
heart (see *Organ Meats*)		
hot dog (see *Luncheon and Deli Meats: frankfurter*)		
kidney (see *Organ Meats*)		
liver (see *Organ Meats*)		
loin		
porterhouse steak		
broiled, lean and fat	3½ oz; ¼" fat trim	25.5
broiled, lean	3½ oz; ¼" fat trim	11.5
T-bone steak		
broiled, lean and fat	3½ oz; ¼" fat trim	23.25
broiled, lean	3½ oz; ¼" fat trim	10
tenderloin		
choice, broiled, lean and fat	3½ oz; ¼" fat trim	21.75
choice, broiled, lean	3½ oz; ¼" fat trim	11.25
prime, broiled, lean and fat	3½ oz; ¼" fat trim	23.5
prime, broiled, lean	3½ oz; ¼" fat trim	12.5

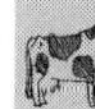
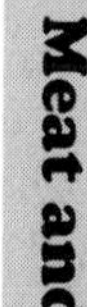

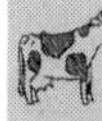

Meat: Beef *(continued)*

Food	Serving Size	Fat
loin *(continued)*		
top sirloin steak		
choice, broiled, lean and fat	3½ oz; ¼" fat trim	16.75
choice, broiled, lean	3½ oz; 0" fat trim	7.75
select, broiled, lean and fat	3½ oz; ¼" fat trim	14
select, broiled, lean	3½ oz; 0" fat trim	5.5

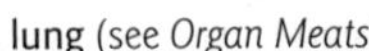

lung (see *Organ Meats*)

pancreas (see *Organ Meats*)

Food	Serving Size	Fat
rib		
whole, choice, roasted, lean and fat	3½ oz; ¼" fat trim	33
whole, choice, roasted, lean	3½ oz; ¼" fat trim	14
whole, prime, roasted, lean and fat	3½ oz; ¼" fat trim	35
whole, prime, roasted, lean	3½ oz; ¼" fat trim	19.5
round		
bottom, choice, braised, lean and fat	3½ oz; ¼" fat trim	18
bottom, choice, braised, lean	3½ oz; 0" fat trim	8.75
bottom, select, braised, lean and fat	3½ oz; ¼" fat trim	15
bottom, select, braised, lean	3½ oz; 0" fat trim	6.75
bottom, choice, roasted, lean and fat	3½ oz; ¼" fat trim	16.5
bottom, choice, roasted, lean	3½ oz; 0" fat trim	7.75
bottom, select, roasted, lean and fat	3½ oz; ¼" fat trim	13.25
bottom, select, roasted, lean	3½ oz; 0" fat trim	5.5
eye, choice, roasted, lean and fat	3½ oz; ¼" fat trim	14
eye, choice, roasted, lean	3½ oz; 0" fat trim	5.75
eye, select, roasted, lean and fat	3½ oz; ¼" fat trim	11.25
eye, select, roasted, lean	3½ oz; 0" fat trim	3.5

Food	Serving Size	Fat

Meat: Beef *(continued)*

Food	Serving Size	Fat
round *(continued)*		
full cut (steak), choice, broiled, lean and fat	3½ oz; ¼" fat trim	13.6
full cut (steak), choice, broiled, lean	3½ oz; ¼" fat trim	7.25
full cut (steak), select, broiled, lean and fat	3½ oz; ¼" fat trim	11.75
full cut (steak), select, broiled, lean	3½ oz; ¼" fat trim	5.25
tip, choice, roasted, lean and fat	3½ oz; ¼" fat trim	15
tip, choice, roasted, lean	3½ oz; 0" fat trim	6.5
tip, prime, roasted, lean and fat	3½ oz; ¼" fat trim	18
tip, prime, roasted, lean	3½ oz; ¼" fat trim	10
top, choice, braised, lean and fat	3½ oz; ¼" fat trim	13
top, choice, braised, lean	3½ oz; 0" fat trim	5.75
top, select, braised, lean and fat	3½ oz; ¼" fat trim	10
top, select, braised, lean	3½ oz; 0" fat trim	4
top, choice, broiled, lean and fat	3½ oz; ¼" fat trim	10.5
top, choice, broiled, lean	3½ oz; ¼" fat trim	6
top, prime, broiled, lean and fat	3½ oz; ¼" fat trim	10.75
top, prime, broiled, lean	3½ oz; ¼" fat trim	9
salami (see *Luncheon and Deli Meats*)		
shank		
choice, simmered, lean and fat	3½ oz; ¼" fat trim	14.75
choice, simmered, lean	3½ oz; ¼" fat trim	6.5
short ribs		
braised, lean and fat	3½ oz	42
braised, lean	3½ oz	18
spleen (see *Organ Meats*)		

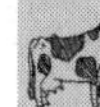
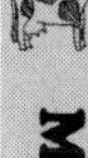
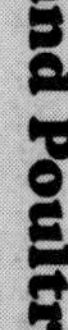

Food	Serving Size	Fat
Meat: Beef *(continued)*		
sweetbreads (see *Organ Meats*)		
tongue (see *Organ Meats*)		
tripe (see *Organ Meats*)		
Meat: Lamb		
brain (see *Organ Meats*)		
cubes		
braised, lean	3½ oz	8.75
broiled, lean	3½ oz	7.25
ground, broiled	3½ oz	19.5
heart (see *Organ Meats*)		
kidney (see *Organ Meats*)		
leg		
roasted, lean and fat	3½ oz	16.5
roasted, lean	3½ oz	7.75
liver (see *Organ Meats*)		
loin		
chop, broiled, lean and fat	3½ oz	23
chop, broiled, lean	3½ oz	9.75
roasted, lean and fat	3½ oz	23.5
roasted, lean	3½ oz	9.75

Food	Serving Size	Fat
Meat: Lamb *(continued)*		
lung (see *Organ Meats*)		
pancreas (see *Organ Meats*)		
rib		
chop, broiled, lean and fat	3½ oz	29.5
chop, broiled, lean	3½ oz	13
roasted, lean and fat	3½ oz	29.75
roasted, lean	3½ oz	13.25
shank		
braised, lean and fat	3½ oz	13.5
braised, lean	3½ oz	6
shoulder		
braised, lean and fat	3½ oz	24.5
braised, lean	3½ oz	16
chop, broiled, lean and fat	3½ oz	19.25
chop, broiled, lean	3½ oz	10.5
roasted, lean and fat	3½ oz	20
roasted, lean	3½ oz	10.75
spleen (see *Organ Meats*)		
tongue (see *Organ Meats*)		

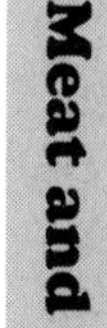

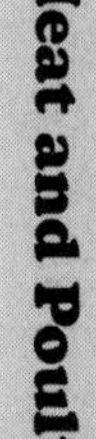

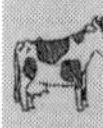

Food	Serving Size	Fat
Meat: Pork		
bacon		
Canadian, grilled	2 slices	4
cured		
raw	2 slices	26
pan fried, broiled	2 slices	6.25
thick sliced, pan fried, broiled	2 slices	10

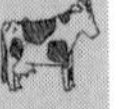

belly (see *Organ Meats*)

bologna (see *Luncheon and Deli Meats*)

brain (see *Organ Meats*)

bratwurst (see *Luncheon and Deli Meats*)

braunschweiger (see *Luncheon and Deli Meats*)

brotwurst (see *Luncheon and Deli Meats*)

chitterlings (see *Organ Meats*)

chorizo (see *Luncheon and Deli Meats*)

ear (see *Organ Meats*)

feet (see *Organ Meats*)

frankfurter (see *Luncheon and Deli Meats*)

Food	Serving Size	Fat
Meat: Pork *(continued)*		
ham (cured)		
roasted	3½ oz	9
canned	3½ oz	13
loaf (see *Luncheon and Deli Meats*)		
patty	2½ oz patty	18.25
steak	3½ oz	4.24
headcheese (see *Luncheon and Deli Meats*)		
heart (see *Organ Meats*)		
hot dog (see *Luncheon and Deli Meats: frankfurter*)		
jowl (see *Organ Meats*)		
kidney (see *Organ Meats*)		
kielbasa (see *Luncheon and Deli Meats*)		
knockwurst (see *Luncheon and Deli Meats*)		
leg		
roasted, lean and fat	3½ oz	17.5
roasted, lean	3½ oz	9.5
liver (see *Organ Meats*)		
liverwurst (see *Luncheon and Deli Meats*)		

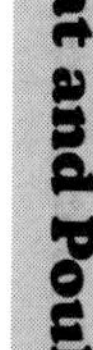

Food	Serving Size	Fat
Meat: Pork *(continued)*		
loin		
braised, lean and fat	3½ oz	13.5
braised, lean	3½ oz	9
broiled, lean and fat	3½ oz	14
broiled, lean	3½ oz	9.75
roasted, lean and fat	3½ oz	14.75
roasted, lean	3½ oz	9.5
braised, lean and fat	3½ oz	25.5
braised, lean	3½ oz	13
broiled, lean and fat	3½ oz	25
broiled, lean	3½ oz	14
loin blade (chop, roast)		
pan fried, lean and fat	3½ oz	27.75
pan fried, lean	3½ oz	15
roasted, lean and fat	3½ oz	24.5
roasted, lean	3½ oz	14.75
lung (see *Organ Meats*)		
pancreas (see *Organ Meats*)		
picnic		
cured, roasted, lean and fat	3½ oz	21.5
cured, roasted, lean	3½ oz	7
braised, lean and fat	3½ oz	23.25
braised, lean	3½ oz	12.25
roasted, lean and fat	3½ oz	24
roasted, lean	3½ oz	12.5
pepperoni (see *Luncheon and Deli Meats*)		

Food	Serving Size	Fat
Meat: Pork *(continued)*		
rib (chop, roast)		
braised, lean and fat	3½ oz	15.75
braised, lean	3½ oz	10
broiled, lean and fat	3½ oz	15.75
broiled, lean	3½ oz	10
pan fried, lean and fat	3½ oz	11.75
pan fried, lean	3½ oz	11.75
roasted, lean and fat	3½ oz	15.25
roasted, lean	3½ oz	10
sparerib, braised	3½ oz	21.5
rolled roast	3½ oz	23.5
rump		
roasted, lean and fat	3½ oz	14.25
roasted, lean	3½ oz	8.25
salami (see *Luncheon and Deli Meats*)		
sausage		
breakfast link, patty	1 oz	8.5
italian	2½ oz	17.25
shank		
roasted, lean and fat	3½ oz	20
roasted, lean	3½ oz	10.5
shoulder		
roasted, lean and fat	3½ oz	21.5
roasted, lean	3½ oz	13.5

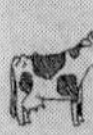

Food	Serving Size	Fat
Meat: Pork *(continued)*		
spleen (see *Organ Meats*)		
stomach (see *Organ Meats*)		
tail (see *Organ Meats*)		
tenderloin		
roasted, lean and fat	3½ oz	6
roasted, lean	3½ oz	4.75
tongue (see *Organ Meats*)		
Meat: Veal		
brain, calf (see *Organ Meats*)		
bockwurst (see *Luncheon and Deli Meats*)		
cubes	3½ oz	4.25
ground, broiled	3½ oz	7.5
heart (see *Organ Meats*)		
kidney (see *Organ Meats*)		
leg		
cutlet, pan fried		
breaded	3½ oz	9.25
not breaded	3½ oz	8.25

Food	Serving Size	Fat
Meat: Veal *(continued)*		
liver, calf (see *Organ Meats*)		
loin		
braised, lean and fat	3½ oz	17.25
braised, lean	3½ oz	9.25
roasted, lean and fat	3½ oz	12.25
roasted, lean	3½ oz	7
lung (see *Organ Meats*)		
pancreas (see *Organ Meats*)		
rib		
braised, lean and fat	3½ oz	12.5
braised, lean	3½ oz	7.75
roasted, lean and fat	3½ oz	14
roasted, lean	3½ oz	7.5
shoulder		
braised, lean and fat	3½ oz	10.25
braised, lean	3½ oz	5.25
roasted, lean and fat	3½ oz	8.25
roasted, lean	3½ oz	5.75
sirloin		
braised, lean and fat	3½ oz	13
braised, lean	3½ oz	6.5
roasted, lean and fat	3½ oz	10.5
roasted, lean	3½ oz	6.25
spleen (see *Organ Meats*)		

Food	Serving Size	Fat
Meat: Veal *(continued)*		
sweetbreads (see *Organ Meats*)		
tongue (see *Organ Meats*)		
Meat: Organ Meats		
belly, pork, raw	1 oz	15
brain		
beef, pan fried	3½ oz	15.75
beef, simmered	3½ oz	12.5
lamb, braised	3½ oz	10.25
lamb, pan fried	3½ oz	22.25
pork, braised	3½ oz	9.5
veal, braised	3½ oz	9.5
veal, pan fried	3½ oz	16.75
chitterlings, pork, simmered	3½ oz	28.75
ear, pork	4 oz; 1 ear	12
feet, pork		
pickled	3½ oz	16
simmered	3½ oz	12.5
smoked hock	3½ oz	13.5
heart		
beef, simmered	3½ oz	5.5
lamb, braised	3½ oz	8
pork, braised	4 ½ oz; 1 heart	6.5
veal, braised	3½ oz	6.75

Food	Serving Size	Fat
Meat: Organ Meats *(continued)*		
jowl, pork, raw	3½ oz	69.5
kidney		
beef, simmered	3½ oz	3.5
lamb, braised	3½ oz	3.5
pork, braised	3½ oz	4.75
veal, braised	3½ oz	5.75
liver		
beef, braised	3½ oz	5
beef, pan fried	3½ oz	8
lamb, braised	3½ oz	8.75
lamb, pan fried	3½ oz	12.75
pork, braised	3½ oz	4.5
veal (calf), braised	3½ oz	7
veal (calf), pan fried	3½ oz	11.5
lung		
beef, braised	3½ oz	3.75
lamb, braised	3½ oz	3
pork, braised	3½ oz	3
veal, braised	3½ oz	2.5
pancreas		
beef, braised	3½ oz	17.25
lamb, braised	3½ oz	15
pork, braised	3½ oz	10.75
veal, braised	3½ oz	14.5
scrapple	1 oz	4

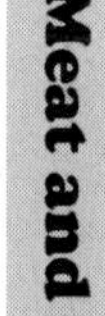

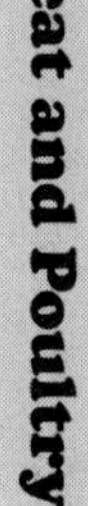

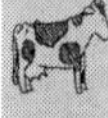

Food	Serving Size	Fat
Meat: Organ Meats *(continued)*		
spleen		
beef, braised	3½ oz	4.25
lamb, braised	3½ oz	4.75
pork, braised	3½ oz	3.25
veal, braised	3½ oz	3
stomach, pork, raw	3½ oz	9.5
sweetbread (thymus)		
beef, braised	3½ oz	25
veal, braised	3½ oz	4.25
tail, pork, simmered	3½ oz	35.75
tongue		
beef, simmered	3½ oz	20.75
lamb, braised	3½ oz	20.25
pork, braised	3½ oz	18.5
veal, braised	3½ oz	10
tripe, raw	3½ oz	4
Poultry: Chicken		
prepared slices, salad (see *Luncheon and Deli Meats*)		
whole, broiler/fryer		
dark meat, with skin		
roasted	3½ oz	15.75
stewed	3½ oz	14.75

Food	Serving Size	Fat
Poultry: Chicken *(continued)*		
whole, broiler/fryer *(continued)*		
dark meat, without skin		
roasted	3½ oz	9.75
stewed	3½ oz	9
light meat, with skin		
roasted	3½ oz	10.75
stewed	3½ oz	10
light meat, without skin		
roasted	3½ oz	4.5
stewed	3½ oz	4
light and dark meat, with skin		
roasted	3½ oz	13.5
stewed	3½ oz	12.5
light and dark meat, without skin		
roasted	3½ oz	7.5
stewed	3½ oz	6.75
whole, capon, with skin, roasted	3½ oz	11.75
whole, roaster		
dark meat, without skin, roasted	3½ oz	8.75
light meat, without skin, roasted	3½ oz	4
dark and light meat, with skin, roasted	3½ oz	13.5
whole, stewer		
dark meat, without skin, stewed	3½ oz	15.25
light meat without skin, stewed	3½ oz	8
light and dark meat, with skin, stewed	3½ oz	19

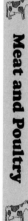

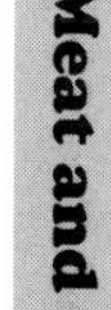

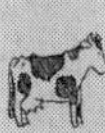

Food	Serving Size	Fat
Poultry: Chicken *(continued)*		
parts		
back, with skin, fried	2½ oz	15
breast, with skin		
fried, flour coated	½ breast	8.75
fried, battered	½ breast	19
roasted	½ breast	7.5
stewed	½ breast	8.25
breast, without skin		
fried, flour coated	½ breast	4
roasted	½ breast	3
stewed	½ breast	3
cutlet (skinless, boneless), raw	4 oz	3
drumstick, with skin (lower leg only)		
fried, flour coated	1; approx 1¾ oz	6.75
fried, battered	1; approx 2½ oz	11
roasted	1; approx 1¾ oz	5.75
stewed	1; approx 1¾ oz	6
leg, with skin (drumstick and thigh)		
fried, flour coated	1; approx 4 oz	16.25
roasted	1; approx 4 oz	15.25
stewed	1; approx 4 oz	16
neck, simmered		
with skin	1 neck	7
without skin	1 neck	1.5
thigh, with skin		
fried, flour coated	1; approx 2 oz	9.25
fried, battered	1; approx 3 oz	14
roasted	1; approx 2 oz	9.5
stewed	1; approx 2 oz	10
thigh, without skin		
roasted	1; approx 2 oz	5.75

Food	Serving Size	Fat

Poultry: Chicken *(continued)*

Food	Serving Size	Fat
parts *(continued)*		
wing, with skin		
fried, flour coated	1; approx 1 oz	7
fried, battered	1; approx 1½ oz	11
roasted	1; approx 1 oz	6.5
stewed	1; approx 1 oz	6.75
spicy	3; approx 3 oz	10
nuggets, breaded	6 pieces; approx 3 oz	19.75
patty	1 patty; approx 2½ oz	11

Poultry: Turkey

prepared breast (see *Luncheon and Deli Meats*)

Food	Serving Size	Fat
whole, roasted		
dark meat, with skin	3½ oz	11.5
dark meat, without skin	3½ oz	7.25
light meat, with skin	3½ oz	8.25
light meat, without skin	3½ oz	3.25
ground, raw	4 oz	10.5
nuggets, breaded	4 pieces; approx 3¼ oz	16
patty, breaded, uncooked	3 oz	13

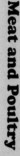

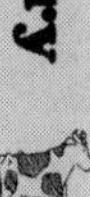

Food	Serving Size	Fat
Poultry: Other		
cornish game hen		
roasted, with skin	½ bird; approx 4 oz	20.75
roasted, without skin	½ bird; approx 4 oz	4.25
duck		
roasted, with skin	3½ oz	28.5
roasted, without skin	3½ oz	11.25
goose		
roasted, with skin	3½ oz	22
roasted, without skin	3½ oz	12.75
pheasant, with skin, raw	3½ oz	9.25
quail, without skin, raw	3½ oz	4.5
Poultry: Organs		
gizzard		
chicken, simmered	3½ oz	3.75
goose, raw	3½ oz	5.25
turkey, simmered	3½ oz	4
heart		
chicken, simmered	3½ oz	8
turkey, simmered	3½ oz	6

Food	Serving Size	Fat
Poultry: Organs *(continued)*		
liver		
chicken, simmered	3½ oz	5.5
duck, raw	3½ oz	4.5
goose, raw	3½ oz	4.5
turkey, simmered	3½ oz	6
Luncheon and Deli Meats*		
beef loaf (lunch meat)	2 oz	7.25
blood sausage (blood pudding)	1 oz	8.5
bockwurst, uncooked	1 link	18
bologna		
beef	1 oz	8.25
light (reduced fat)	1 oz	4
beef and pork	1 oz	8
chicken, pork, and beef	1 oz	8.25
Lebanon	1 oz	3.5
pork	1 oz	5.5
turkey	1 oz	4.25
turkey, beef, and pork, fat free	1 oz	.25
bratwurst	3 oz link	22
braunschweiger	1 oz	8.5
brotwurst	2½ oz link	19.5

*Average fat; fat counts vary widely among brands.

Food	Serving Size	Fat
Luncheon and Deli Meats *(continued)*		
chicken roll	1 oz	3
chorizo	2 oz link	23
corned beef	2 oz	7
frankfurter (hot dog)		
beef	2 oz link; 8 per lb	16.25
fat free	2 oz link; 8 per lb	1.75
beef and pork	2 oz link; 8 per lb	16.5
chicken	1½ oz link; 10 per lb	8.75
pork and turkey	1½ oz link; 10 per lb	13.5
pork, turkey, and beef, light	2 oz link; 8 per lb	8.5
turkey	1½ oz link; 10 per lb	8
turkey and beef, fat free	1¾ oz link	.25
turkey and chicken	1½ oz link; 10 per lb	5.75
turkey, chicken, and beef, fat free	2 oz link; 8 per lb	2
ham and cheese		
loaf	1 oz	5
spread	1 oz	5.25

Food	Serving Size	Fat
Luncheon and Deli Meats *(continued)*		
ham, deli style (also see *Meat: Pork*)		
baked	2 oz	1.5
boiled	2 oz	2
deviled	⅓ cup; 3 oz	18
glazed	2 oz	1.5
minced, loaf	2 oz	11.5
salad spread	1 oz	4.5
smoked	2 oz	2
turkey	2 oz	3
headcheese	1 oz	4.5
hot dog (see *frankfurter*)		
kielbasa	1 oz	7.25
knockwurst	1 oz	7.75
liver pâté		
chicken	1 oz	3.75
goose (foie gras)	1 oz	12.5
liverwurst	1 oz	8
mortadella	2 oz	14
olive loaf	1 oz	4.5
pastrami		
beef	1 oz	2
turkey	1 oz	1.75

Food	Serving Size	Fat
Luncheon and Deli Meats *(continued)*		
pepperoni	1 oz	13.25
pimento loaf	1 oz	6
salami		
beef	1 oz	5
beef and pork	1 oz	5
cooked (cotto)		
beef, chicken, and pork	1 oz	5.5
beef	1 oz	4.25
turkey	1 oz	2.75
dry/hard		
pork	1 oz	9.5
pork and beef	1 oz	9.5
genoa	1 oz	9
turkey	1 oz	2.75
smoked link sausage		
beef	1½ oz link	11.5
pork	2½ oz link	21.5
pork and beef	2½ oz link	20.5
pork and turkey	2 oz link	15
thuringer		
beef and pork	1 oz	7
beef	1 oz	7.5
turkey breast		
roasted		
fat free	2 oz	.5
with skin	3½ oz	3.5

Food	Serving Size	Fat
Luncheon and Deli Meats *(continued)*		
turkey breast *(continued)*		
smoked	1 oz	1
fat free	2 oz	.5
turkey ham (see *ham*)		
turkey pastrami (see *pastrami*)		
turkey salami (see *salami*)		
Vienna sausage		
reduced fat		
25%	1.9 oz; 3 links	11
50%	1.9 oz; 3 links	7
beef and pork	1¾ oz; 3 links	12
chicken	1¾ oz; 3 links	8
in barbecue sauce	2 oz; 3 links and sauce	12
smoked	2 oz; 3 links	14
Meat and Poultry Substitutes*		
bacon		
strips	½ oz; 2 strips	5
bits	1½ tbsp	1
bean/lentil loaf	3 oz	8

*Average fat; fat counts vary widely among brands.

Meat and Poultry Substitutes *(continued)*

Food	Serving Size	Fat
breakfast sausage		
links	1 oz; 1 link	4.5
patty	1⅓ oz; 1 patty	7
burger	2 oz	2
"chicken"		
nuggets	3 oz; 5 pieces	16
patty	2½ oz	9.75
frankfurter	2 oz; 1 piece	6.75
meat extender	1 oz	.75

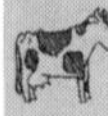

Food	Serving Size	Fat
Nuts*		
almonds		
whole, chopped, slivered	1 oz	14.5
dry roasted	1 oz	14.5
oil roasted	1 oz	16
honey roasted	1 oz	14
barbecue flavor	1 oz	15
meal	1 oz	5.25
butter	1 tbsp	9.5
paste	1 oz	8
brazil nuts	1 oz	18.75
cashews		
dry roasted	1 oz	13
oil roasted	1 oz	13.75
honey roasted	1 oz	13
butter	1 oz	14
chestnuts, fresh, roasted	1 oz	.5
water chestnuts (see *Vegetables*)		
coconut		
fresh	1 oz	9.5
dried, shredded		
sweetened	1 cup	33
unsweetened	1 oz	18
cream, sweetened	1 cup	52.5
milk	1 cup	57.25
water	1 cup	.5

*Edible portion only (no shells), unless otherwise indicated.

Food	Serving Size	Fat
Nuts *(continued)*		
filberts (see *hazelnuts)*		
hazelnuts		
whole	1 oz	15.5
chopped, sliced	1 oz	14.5
dry roasted	1 oz	18.75
oil roasted	1 oz	18
butter	1 tbsp	10
with chocolate (Nutella)	1 tbsp	4.5
hickory	1 oz	18.25
macadamia		
dry roasted	1 oz	21
oil roasted	1 oz	21.75
mixed		
dry roasted	1 oz	16
honey roasted	1 oz	13
oil roasted	1 oz	16
peanuts		
raw	1 oz	14
dry roasted	1 oz	14
honey roasted	1 oz	11
roasted in oil	1 oz	14
Spanish		
raw	1 oz	14
oil roasted	1 oz	14

Food	Serving Size	Fat
Nuts *(continued)*		
peanut butter*		
creamy, smooth	2 tbsp	16.25
chunky	2 tbsp	16
reduced fat	2 tbsp	12
with jelly	2 tbsp	10
pecans		
halves	1 oz	19.25
chopped	½ cup	30
oil roasted	1 oz	20.25
honey roasted	1 oz	18
pine nuts (pignoli)	1 oz	14.5
pistachios		
in shells	2 oz	14
shelled	1 oz	13.75
soy nuts		
dry roasted	1 oz	6
oil roasted	1 oz	7
walnuts		
whole, halves	1 oz	19
chopped	1 cup	72
ground	½ cup	24

*Average fat; fat counts vary widely among brands.

Food	Serving Size	Fat
Seeds*		
flax	1 oz	10
pumpkin	1 oz	13
sesame		
raw	1 tbsp	4.5
toasted	1 oz	13.5
tahini (sesame paste)		
raw	1 tbsp	8
toasted	1 tbsp	8
sunflower		
raw	1 oz	14
toasted	1 oz	16
dry roasted	1 oz	14
oil roasted	1 oz	16.25

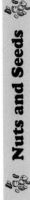

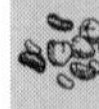

*See *Extras: Herbs and Spices* for herb and spice seeds.

Food	Serving Size	Fat

Note: Except for brand names, average fat; fat counts vary widely among brands.

Chips and Nibbles

Food	Serving Size	Fat
banana chips	1 oz	7
beef stick, smoked	½ oz stick	4
beef jerky	.7 oz piece	5
Bugles	1½ cup	9
carrot chips	1 oz	9
cheese balls, curls	1 oz	10
reduced fat	1 oz	5
cheese puffs	1 oz	9.75
cheese straws	5 pieces; approx 1 oz	9
Chex mix	1 oz	4.75
corn chips		
plain	1 oz	9.5
nacho	1 oz	7
tortilla	1 oz	7.5

Cracker Jack (see *popcorn, caramel coated*)

crackers (see *Breads, Crackers, and Baked Goods)*

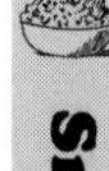

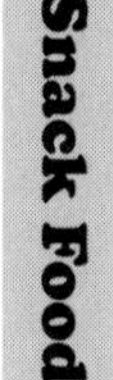

Food	Serving Size	Fat
Chips and Nibbles *(continued)*		
Goldfish	1 oz	6
mix, snack, party	1 oz	10
oriental	1 oz	7.5
popcorn		
kernels, unpopped	1/4 cup	2.5
air popped (no fat added)	1 oz; approx 3½ cups	0
oil popped	1 oz; approx 3½ cups	3
microwave		
buttered	1 oz; approx 3½ cups	2
light	1 oz; approx 3½ cups	1
bagged	1 oz; approx 3½ cups	10
movie theater		
small	approx 7 cups	27
buttered	approx 7 cups	47
medium	approx 16 cups	60
buttered	approx 16 cups	90
large	approx 20 cups	76
buttered	approx 20 cups	116
caramel coated	1 oz	2
pork rinds	1 oz	9

Food	Serving Size	Fat
Chips and Nibbles *(continued)*		
potato chips		
plain	1 oz	9.75
reduced fat	1 oz	6
no fat (made with Olestra)	1 oz	0
flavored (barbecue, onion, garlic, sour cream and onion, etc.)	1 oz	9
cheese	1 oz	7.75
sweet potato	1 oz	7
potato sticks	1 oz	9.75
pretzels		
regular	1 oz	1
chocolate coated	1 oz	4.75
soft	2½ oz	0
rice cakes *(see Breads, Crackers, and Baked Goods)*		
vegetable chips	1 oz	4
Dips and Spreads		
avocado (guacamole)	2 tbsp	5
baba gannouj (eggplant/tahini)	2 tbsp	6
bean	2 tbsp	1
blue cheese	2 tbsp	7
cheese	2 tbsp	7

Food	Serving Size	Fat
Dips and Spreads *(continued)*		
clam	2 tbsp	4.5
hummus (chickpeas/tahini)	2 tbsp	1
jalapeño	2 tbsp	1
nacho	2 tbsp	4
pâté (also see *Meat and Poultry: Luncheon and Deli Meats*)		
smoked salmon	1 oz	3.5
spinach	1 oz	4
salsa	2 tbsp	0
sour cream–onion		
regular	2 tbsp	4
low fat	2 tbsp	2
sour cream–onion-bacon, regular	2 tbsp	5
spinach	2 tbsp	6
taramasalata (fish roe)		
regular	1 tbsp	10
light	1 tbsp	4
vegetable	2 tbsp	0
yogurt-cucumber (tzatziki)	2 tbsp	3

Food	Serving Size	Fat
Energy Bars		
breakfast	1⅓ oz bar	2.5
granola	1⅓ oz bar	2.75
fruit	1⅓ oz bar	2
low fat	1 oz bar	2
peanut butter	1 oz bar	4.5
Sweet Snacks: Candy*		
bars		
Almond Joy	1.7 oz bar	13
Baby Ruth	2.1 oz bar	12.75
Bit-O-Honey	1.7 oz bar	3.75
Butterfinger	2.16 oz bar	11.5
Charleston Chew	1.9 oz bar	7
Fifth Avenue	2 oz bar	8.5
Heath	1.4 oz bar	13
Kit Kat	1.5 oz bar	11.25
Mars	1.8 oz bar	11.5
Milky Way	2.15 oz bar	9.75
Mounds	1.9 oz bar	13.25
Mr. Goodbar	1¾ oz bar	15.75
Nestlé Crunch	1.4 oz bar	10.5
Oh Henry!	2 oz bar	9.5
Snickers	2.16 oz bar	15
Three Musketeers	2.13 oz bar	7.75

*Except for brand name items, average fat; fat counts vary widely among brands. Read the label and pay attention to serving size as packaged sizes vary widely.

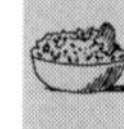

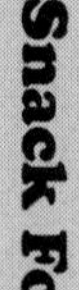

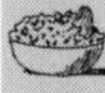

Food	Serving Size	Fat
Sweet Snacks: Candy *(continued)*		
bits		
after dinner mints	1 piece	.5
butterscotch	1 oz	1
candy corn	1 oz	0
caramel	2½ oz	5.75
chocolate-covered (see *chocolate*)		
Good & Plenty	1 oz	0
Good & Fruity	1 oz	.5
gumdrops	1 oz	0
gummies	1⅓ oz	0
hard candy (sour balls)	1 oz	0
sugar free	1 oz	0
jelly beans	1 oz	tr
jordan almonds (candy coated)	1 oz	5.25
Life Savers	1 piece	0
licorice (see *licorice*)		
M&Ms		
regular	1.69 oz bag	10
peanut	1.74 oz bag	13
malted milk balls	1⅓ oz	6
maple sugar candy	1 oz	tr
mint lozenges	1 oz	.5
Necco wafers	2 oz	0
nougat	1 oz	1
Now and Later	1 pkg	.5
Peppermint Patties	1½ oz	3
Reese's Peanut Butter Cups	1.8 oz	17
Reese's Pieces	1.6 oz	9.75
saltwater taffy	1 oz	1
spearmint leaves (see *gumdrops*)		
Skittles	2⅓ oz	2.75

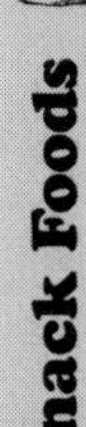

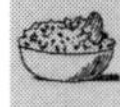

Food	Serving Size	Fat
Sweet Snacks: Candy *(continued)*		
bits *(continued)*		
Starburst	2.07 oz	5
Tic Tac	1 piece	0
toffee	½ oz	4
Tootsie Rolls	1 piece	.5
bubble gum (see *gum*)		
candy cane	½ oz	0
carob		
bar	1 oz	9
carob-coated nuts	1 oz	10
carob-coated raisins	1 oz	5
chewing gum (see *gum*)		
chocolate		
baking (see *Sweets and Desserts: Baking Ingredients*)		
dark	1 oz	10
with nuts	1 oz	12.5
milk	1 oz	10
with nuts	1 oz	12.5
fudge	1 oz	2.25
with nuts	1 oz	4.5
chocolate coffee beans	1 oz	7
chocolate-covered cherry	1	2
chocolate-covered mints	1 oz	2
chocolate-covered nuts	1 oz	12.5
chocolate-covered raisins	1 oz	3.5
with filled centers	1 oz	5

Food	Serving Size	Fat
Sweet Snacks: Candy *(continued)*		
chocolate *(continued)*		
Hershey's Kisses	1 oz	12.5
truffles	½ oz	4
cough drops	1 drop	0
fruit leather/rolls	1 oz	2
fruit peel (see *Fruits: citrus peel*)		
gum, all types	1 stick	0
halvah	1 oz	12.5
licorice, all types	1 oz	0
lollipops, all types	1 lollipop	0
marshmallows	1 piece	0
marzipan	1 oz	7
peanut brittle	1 oz	5.5
praline	1 oz	6.75
sesame bar	1 oz	9.25
trail mix	2 oz	7
yogurt-covered raisins	1 oz	4

Food	Serving Size	Fat
Note: For home recipes, use values for individual ingredients to determine total fat.		
Soups*		
asparagus, cream of		
canned, reconstituted		
made with milk	1 cup	8.25
made with water	1 cup	4
made from mix	1 cup	1.75
bean		
black, canned, reconstituted	1 cup	1.5
with bacon		
canned, reconstituted	1 cup	6
made from mix	1 cup	2
with franks, canned, reconstituted	1 cup	7
beef		
bouillon, cube or powder	1 cube or 1 tsp	0
broth	1 cup	0
consommé	1 cup	0
tomato beef noodle	1 cup	4.25
with mushrooms	1 cup	3
with noodles		
canned, reconstituted	1 cup	3
made from mix	1 cup	.75

*Average fat; fat counts vary widely among brands. Fat counts are based on a 1-cup serving; many containers hold more than one serving, so read the label.

Food	Serving Size	Fat
Soups *(continued)*		
beef *(continued)*		
with vegetables, canned	1 cup	3.75
fat free	1 cup	2
and barley, canned, reconstituted	1 cup	2
borscht	1 cup	0
broccoli		
cream of		
canned, reconstituted	1 cup	6
fat free	1 cup	4
with cheese	1 cup	7
fat free	1 cup	2.5
cauliflower, made from mix	1 cup	1.75
celery, cream of		
canned, reconstituted		
made with milk	1 cup	9.75
made with water	1 cup	5.5
made from mix	1 cup	1.5
cheese		
canned, reconstituted		
made with milk	1 cup	14.5
made with water	1 cup	10.5
chicken		
bouillon, cube or powder	1 cube or 1 tsp	0
broth	1 cup	1.5
fat free	1 cup	0

Food	Serving Size	Fat
Soups *(continued)*		
chicken *(continued)*		
cream of, canned, reconstituted		
made with milk	1 cup	11.5
made with water	1 cup	7.5
made from mix	1 cup	5.25
gumbo, canned, reconstituted	1 cup	1.5
with dumplings, canned, reconstituted	1 cup	5.5
with matzo balls, home recipe	1 cup	7
with noodles		
canned, reconstituted	1 cup	2.5
fat free	1 cup	1.25
made from mix	1 cup	1.25
with rice		
canned, reconstituted	1 cup	2
made from mix	1 cup	1.5
with vegetables		
canned, reconstituted	1 cup	2.75
made from mix	1 cup	.75
clam chowder		
Manhattan style		
canned, reconstituted	1 cup	2.25
made from mix	1 cup	1.5
New England style		
canned, reconstituted		
made with milk	1 cup	6.5
made with water	1 cup	5
made from mix	1 cup	3.75
french onion (see *onion*)		

Food	Serving Size	Fat
Soups *(continued)*		
gazpacho	1 cup	.25
leek, made from mix	1 cup	2
lentil		
canned, reconstituted	1 cup	.5
fat free	1 cup	1.25
made from mix	1 cup	1
minestrone		
canned, reconstituted	1 cup	2.5
fat free	1 cup	1.25
made from mix	1 cup	1.75
mushroom		
canned, reconstituted	1 cup	4
made from mix	1 cup	5
cream of		
canned, reconstituted		
made with milk	1 cup	13.5
made with water	1 cup	9
made from mix	6 oz	2
with barley	1 cup	2.25
onion		
canned, reconstituted	1 cup	1.75
cream of		
made with milk	1 cup	9.5
made with water	1 cup	5.25
made from mix	1 cup	.5

Food	Serving Size	Fat
Soups *(continued)*		
oyster stew, canned, reconstituted		
made with milk	1 cup	8
made with water	1 cup	3.75
pasta e fagioli, home recipe	1 cup	5
pea, split		
canned, reconstituted		
made with milk	1 cup	7
made with water	1 cup	3
with ham, made with water	1 cup	4.5
made from mix	1 cup	1.5
pepperpot, canned, reconstituted	1 cup	5
potato, cream of		
canned, reconstituted		
made with milk	1 cup	6.5
made with water	1 cup	2.5
ramen noodle		
beef	2 oz pkg	11
chicken	2 oz pkg	11
pork	1½ oz pkg	6
shrimp	1½ oz pkg	6
scotch broth, canned, reconstituted	1 cup	2.5

Food	Serving Size	Fat
Soups *(continued)*		
shrimp, cream of		
canned, reconstituted		
made with milk	1 cup	9.25
made with water	1 cup	5.25
tomato, canned, reconstituted		
made with milk	1 cup	6
made with water	1 cup	2
made from mix	1 cup	2.5
bisque		
made with milk	1 cup	6.5
made with water	1 cup	2.5
with rice	1 cup	2.75
vegetable	1 cup	.5
turkey		
with noodles	1 cup	2
with vegetables	1 cup	3
vegetable		
bouillon, cube or powder	1 cube or 1 tsp	0
broth	1 cup	0
with beef, canned, reconstituted	1 cup	2
fat free	1 cup	2
vegetarian	1 cup	2
vichyssoise (see *potato, cream of*)		
wonton	1 cup	7

Food	Serving Size	Fat
Packaged Entrées*		
Hamburger Helper (as prepared, with ground beef)		
Beef Romanoff	1 cup	11
Beef Stew	1 cup	10
Cheddar Primavera	1 cup	14
Cheeseburger Macaroni	1 cup	16
Cheesy Italian	1 cup	14
Chili Macaroni	1 cup	10
Hamburger Stew	1 cup	10
Lasagna	1 cup	10
Meat Loaf	1 cup	15
Nacho Cheese	1 cup	13
Potatoes au Gratin	1 cup	14
Salisbury	1 cup	10
Stroganoff	1 cup	13
Swedish Meatball	1 cup	14
Zesty Italian	1 cup	11
Zesty Mexican	1 cup	11
Pizzas** (frozen)		
cheese	3½ oz	12
combination	3½ oz	13.5
pepperoni	3½ oz	13.5
sausage	3½ oz	12.75
French bread style		
cheese	5¾ oz	15.75

*No attempt has been made to include all packaged and frozen entrées since full nutritional information is available on the label. Except for brand name items, average fat; fat counts vary widely among brands and recipes. Fat counts are based on a 1-cup serving; many containers hold more than one serving.

*Average fat; fat counts vary widely among brands and recipes.

Food	Serving Size	Fat
Packaged Entrées *(continued)*		
Pizzas (frozen) *(continued)*		
French bread style *(continued)*		
pepperoni	6 oz	20
sausage	6¼ oz	15.75
Lean Cuisine		
cheese	5 oz	9
pepperoni	5½ oz	12
sausage	6 oz	10
Pot Pies*		
beef	1 pie; approx 7 oz	17
chicken	1 pie; approx 7 oz	20
turkey	1 pie; approx 7 oz	20.5
vegetable cheese	1 pie; approx 7 oz	18
Tuna Helper (as prepared with canned tuna)		
Au Gratin	1 cup	12
Cheesy Pasta	1 cup	11
Creamy Broccoli	1 cup	12
Creamy Pasta	1 cup	13
Garden Cheddar	1 cup	12
Tetrazzini	1 cup	12
Tuna Romanoff	1 cup	8

*Average fat; fat counts vary widely among brands and recipes.

Food	Serving Size	Fat
Mexican Specialties*		
burrito		
bean and cheese	1; approx 3 oz	6
beef	1; approx 4 oz	10
chicken	1; approx 4 oz	4
chili		
beans only	1 cup	8
con carne	1 cup	14
meat only	1 cup	28
enchilada		
beef	5.7 oz	6
cheese	5.7 oz	4
fajita (fast food style)		
chicken	1; approx 8 oz	21
steak	1; approx 8 oz	21.25
menudo	1 cup	3
nachos	approx 3½ oz	18
quesadilla	1	10
taco	1; approx 6 oz	20.5
tamale	2; approx 6 oz	20.75
tostada (beef, beans, cheese)	1; approx 8 oz	17

*Average fat; fat counts vary widely among brands and recipes.

Food	Serving Size	Fat
Noodle Dishes*		
beef and noodles	1 cup	8
beef stroganoff	1 cup	27
chicken and noodles	1 cup	18.5
chow mein	1 cup	10
noodles romanoff	3 oz	7
tuna noodle casserole	6 oz	9.5
turkey tetrazzini	6 oz	14.5
Pasta Dishes*		
pasta (all shapes)		
with broccoli and cheese	1 cup	5.25
with cheddar	1 cup	4
with three cheese	1 cup	6.5
with four cheese	1 cup	6
with marinara sauce	8 oz	6.5
with meatballs	1 cup	11.75
with meat sauce	1 cup	10
primavera	8 oz	12
with oil and garlic	1 cup	16
with pesto sauce	1 cup	14
with sausage and tomato sauce	8 oz	13
with tomato sauce	1 cup	8.75
salad	8 oz	7

*Average fat; fat counts vary widely among brands and recipes.

Food	Serving Size	Fat
Pasta Dishes *(continued)*		
cannelloni	6 oz	15
fettucine Alfredo	8 oz	19
gnocchi, with tomato sauce	8 oz	18
lasagna, with meat and tomato sauce	8 oz	15.5
macaroni and cheese	1 cup	10
manicotti with cheese and tomato sauce	8 oz	14
ravioli, beef with sauce	8 oz	12
tortellini, cheese with tomato sauce	5½ oz	9
Rice Dishes*		
fried rice (Chinese)	1 cup	2
pilaf	½ cup	1.5
risotto	1 cup	18
Spanish rice	½ cup	4.5
white and wild rice pilaf	½ cup	2
yellow rice (Mexican)	½ cup	3.5

*Average fat; fat counts vary widely among brands and recipes.

Food	Serving Size	Fat
Stews*		
beef and vegetable	1 cup	7.5
beef burgundy	7½ oz	18.5
bouillabaise	1 cup	7.5
Brunswick stew	1 cup	6.25
chicken à la king	1 cup	34.25
chicken and dumplings	7 oz	14
chicken cacciatore	7 oz	10
chicken fricassee	1 cup	22.25
chipped beef, creamed	1 cup	25.25
moussaka	8 oz	22
osso buco (excluding bones)	8 oz	28
oyster stew	1 cup	15.5
pot roast beef	7½ oz	6
Miscellaneous*		
cheese fondue	½ cup	14.5

*Average fat; fat counts vary widely among brands and recipes.

Food	Serving Size	Fat
Miscellaneous *(continued)*		
corned beef hash	1 cup	30
crab cake	1 piece; approx 2 oz	4.5
croquettes		
chicken, with gravy	2 pieces; approx 5¾ oz	20
ham	1 piece; approx 2½ oz	10
dolmas (stuffed grape leaves)	3 pieces	5
egg roll (Chinese)	1 piece; approx 3 oz	6
escargots (snails), garlic butter	6	10
falafel	3 pieces; approx 3 oz	9.5
fish loaf	1 slice; approx 5 oz	6
fish patty	1 piece; approx 3 oz	12
fritters		
clam	1 piece; approx 1¼ oz	6

Food	Serving Size	Fat
Miscellaneous *(continued)*		
fritters *(continued)*		
corn	1 piece; approx 1 oz	7.25
frog legs (raw, meat only)	4 oz	.25
meat loaf	1 slice; approx 3 oz	7.75
quiche		
Lorraine	1 piece; approx 3 oz	32
spinach and mushroom	1 piece; approx 3 oz	15
soufflé		
cheese	1 cup	16.25
spinach	1 cup	18.5
stuffed cabbage (with beef and rice)	1 piece; approx 7 oz	10
stuffed pepper (with beef and rice)	1 piece; approx 6½ oz	10
spanakopita	3 oz	19
veal marsala	8 oz	15
veal parmigiana	8 oz	20
Welsh rarebit	1 cup	31

Food	Serving Size	Fat
Baking ingredients		
baking powder	1 tsp	0
baking soda	1 tsp	0
Bisquick		
regular	1 cup	18
reduced fat	1 cup	7.5
chocolate		
unsweetened	1 oz	15
semisweet	1 oz	8
white	1 oz	9
chips		
semisweet	1 oz	6
mint	1 oz	8.5
peanut butter	1 oz	8.5
white	1 oz	4
cocoa powder	1 tbsp	.75
cornstarch	1 tbsp	0
cream of tartar	1 tsp	0
flour (also see *Cereals, Grains, Pasta, and Rice*)		
arrowroot	1 cup	tr
buckwheat	1 cup	3.75
carob	1 cup	.75
corn	1 cup	4.25
potato	1 cup	1.5
rice, brown	1 cup	4.5

Food	Serving Size	Fat
Baking ingredients *(continued)*		
flour (also see *Cereals, Grains, Pasta, and Rice*) *(continued)*		
rice, white	1 cup	2.25
rye, dark	1 cup	3.5
rye, medium	1 cup	1.75
rye, light	1 cup	1.5
self rising	1 cup	1.25
semolina	1 cup	2
soy	1 cup	6
low fat	1 cup	6
white	1 cup	1.25
whole wheat	1 cup	2.25
graham cracker crumbs	1 cup	11.5
pie crust (see *Pies, Fillings, and Crusts*)		
yeast	¼ oz pkg	.25
Cakes*		
angel food	1 oz; 1/12 cake	.25
apple crumb	2 oz	10
banana, frosted	2½ oz	19
black forest	1½ oz	22

*Average fat; fat counts vary widely among brands and recipes.
Unless otherwise noted, cakes are without icing; for iced cake, add fat value of 2 tbsp or 1 oz icing per serving.

Food	Serving Size	Fat
Cakes *(continued)*		
brownie	1 piece; 2 oz	9
with nuts	1 piece; 2 oz	9
bundt	3 oz slice	17
carrot		
plain	2½ oz slice	11
with cream cheese icing	2½ oz slice	21
cheese		
plain	2¾ oz slice	18
with fruit topping	5 oz slice	26.25
low fat	3 oz slice	8
chocolate		
plain	3½ oz slice	14.25
with frosting	4 oz slice	20
pudding-style	2¾ oz slice	14.25
fat free	1½ oz slice	0
cinnamon crumb	4 oz slice	23
coconut, with icing	3 oz slice	21
coffee	2 oz slice	14.75
cupcake		
with chocolate icing	1¾ oz	6.5
with white icing	1¾ oz	5.5

Food	Serving Size	Fat
Cakes *(continued)*		
devil's food		
plain	1½ oz slice	5
with chocolate icing	3 oz slice	15
reduced fat	1½ oz slice	7
fruit	1½ oz piece	4
gingerbread	2½ oz piece	12
lemon	2¾ oz slice	11
chiffon	2 oz slice	3
fat free	1½ oz slice	0
pudding-style	3 oz slice	4
with poppy seeds	3 oz slice	12
marble	2½ oz slice	12.5
pineapple upside down	4 oz piece	14
pound	2 oz slice	13
snack cakes		
Devil Dog	1½ oz	7
Ding Dong	1 piece; approx 1½ oz	9
Drake's coffee cake	1 oz	6
Ho-Ho	1 piece; 1 oz	6
Ring-Ding	1 piece; approx 1½ oz	9
Sno Ball	1; approx 1¾ oz	5
Tastykake low fat lemon cupcake	1 piece; 1 oz	1

Food	Serving Size	Fat
Cakes *(continued)*		
snack cakes *(continued)*		
Twinkies	2 pieces; 1½ oz	5
light	2 pieces; 1½ oz	2.5
Yodels	1 piece; approx 1 oz	16
spice	3 oz slice	11
sponge	2 oz slice	2.75
tiramisu	4 oz piece	23.25
white	2½ oz slice	9.25
with coconut icing	4 oz slice	11.5
reduced fat	1½ oz slice	6
yellow	2½ oz slice	10
with chocolate icing	3½ oz slice	17
with white icing	3½ oz slice	14.5
light	1 oz slice	1.5
pudding-style	2½ oz slice	11
Cake Frostings, Icings, and Fillings*		
butter cream	2 tbsp	5
butterscotch	2 tbsp	5
caramel	2 tbsp	5

*Average fat; fat counts vary widely among brands and recipes.

Food	Serving Size	Fat
Cake Frostings, Icings, and Fillings *(continued)*		
cake and cookie decoration		
chocolate	1 tbsp	1.75
all other flavors	1 tbsp	2
chocolate		
home recipe, creamy	2 tbsp	2.75
home recipe, glaze	2 tbsp	2
ready made, creamy	2 tbsp	4.75
low fat	2 tbsp	1
cream filling (boiled)	½ cup	7
cream cheese	2 tbsp	6.5
fudge	2 tbsp	6
lemon	2 tbsp	5
mocha, ready made	2 tbsp	5
sour cream	2 tbsp	6.5
sugar icing/glaze, home recipe	2 tbsp	2
vanilla		
home recipe	2 tbsp	2
ready made	2 tbsp	6
light	2 tbsp	2
white, boiled, home recipe	2 tbsp	0

Food	Serving Size	Fat
Candy *(see Snack Foods: Sweet Snacks)*		
Cookies*		
almond	1 oz	7
anisette	1 oz	0
biscotti	1 oz	4
butter	1 oz	5
chocolate	1 oz	7
mint	1 oz	7
chocolate chip		
small	½ oz	3
medium	1 oz	6
large	2½ oz	14
jumbo	4 oz	22
with nuts	1 oz	7
reduced fat	1 oz	5
coconut, chocolate covered	1 oz	9
fortune (Chinese)	1 cookie	.25
fudge	1 oz	7

*Average fat; fat counts vary widely among brands and recipes. Cookie sizes also vary widely; for packaged cookies, read the label.

Food	Serving Size	Fat
Cookies *(continued)*		
ginger snaps	4 cookies; approx 1 oz	2.5
graham crackers	5 pieces; 1 oz	3
low fat	4 pieces; approx 1 oz	1.5
chocolate covered	1 oz	6.5
hazelnut	4 pieces; 1 oz	9
lady fingers	1 piece	1
lemon	1 oz	5
macaroons	1 oz	6
marshmallow, chocolate covered	2 pieces; 1 oz	5
molasses	1 oz	3.5
newtons		
fig	2 pieces; 1 oz	2.5
fat free	2 pieces; 1 oz	0
other fruit	2 pieces; 1 oz	0
oatmeal, with raisins		
small	½ oz	1.5
medium	1 oz	3.5
large	2½ oz	9
fat free	1 oz	.4

Food	Serving Size	Fat
Cookies *(continued)*		
peanut butter	2 cookies; 1 oz	3
refrigerated cookie dough		
chocolate	1 oz	6
chocolate chip	1 oz	6
oatmeal	1 oz	6
peanut butter	1 oz	6
sugar	1 oz	5
sandwich		
chocolate covered	1 cookie; approx ¾ oz	6
cream filled, chocolate	2 cookies; approx 1½ oz	7
double filled	2 cookies; 1 oz	7
reduced fat	3 cookies; approx 1 oz	3.5
cream filled, peanut butter	2 cookies; 1 oz	6
cream filled, vanilla	3 cookies; approx 1 oz	6
reduced fat	1 oz	4.5
shortbread	1 oz	7
shortcake	1 oz	3.5
sugar	1 oz	7
vanilla wafers	1 oz	7
reduced fat	1 oz	2

Food	Serving Size	Fat
Cookies *(continued)*		
waffle	1 oz	10
Frozen Desserts: Ice Cream, Ices, Yogurts, Sorbets*		
Cones**		
sugar	1	.5
waffle	1	1
Ice Cream		
banana nut	½ cup	9
butter pecan	½ cup	12
cherry vanilla	½ cup	8
chocolate	½ cup	10
low fat	½ cup	5
chocolate chip	½ cup	14
fudge	½ cup	16
bar, with chocolate coating	3½ oz bar	24.75

*Average fat; fat counts vary widely among brands. Butterfat content of ice creams run from 0% (fat free), 4% (low fat), 6% (reduced fat) to 10% (regular) and 16%–20% for premium. This affects both calorie and fat counts. Read the label.

**Single scoops are generally 3 oz. Add ice cream portion to unfilled cone to obtain total fat.

Food	Serving Size	Fat
Frozen Desserts: Ice Cream, Ices, Yogurts, Sorbets *(continued)*		
Ice Cream *(continued)*		
chocolate chip	½ cup	10
mint	½ cup	10
light	½ cup	5
cookie dough	½ cup	10
coffee	½ cup	10
low fat	½ cup	.5
macadamia nut brittle	½ cup	20
Neapolitan	½ cup	9
low fat	½ cup	4
peach	½ cup	6
low fat	½ cup	.5
pecan praline	½ cup	11
peppermint	½ cup	8
pistachio	½ cup	10
rocky road	½ cup	9
rum raisin	½ cup	17
low fat	½ cup	.5
sandwich	1	13

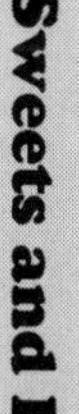

Food	Serving Size	Fat
Frozen Desserts: Ice Cream, Ices, Yogurts, Sorbets *(continued)*		
Ice Cream *(continued)*		
strawberry	½ cup	6
low fat	½ cup	.25
vanilla	½ cup	9
low fat	½ cup	4
cookies and cream	½ cup	9
low fat	½ cup	2.25
fudge	½ cup	8
fat free	½ cup	0
Swiss almond	½ cup	21
bar, with chocolate coating	3½ oz bar	22.5
bar, with chocolate and almond coating	3½ oz bar	23
Tofu-Based		
berry	½ cup	9
"butter" pecan	½ cup	13
chocolate	½ cup	11
cookie crunch	½ cup	11
vanilla	½ cup	11
fudge	½ cup	9
Frozen Yogurt		
hard, all flavors		
low fat	½ cup	3
nonfat	½ cup	0

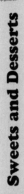

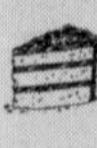

Food	Serving Size	Fat

Frozen Desserts: Ice Cream, Ices, Yogurts, Sorbets
(continued)

Food	Serving Size	Fat
Frozen Yogurt *(continued)*		
soft, all flavors		
lowfat	½ cup	2.5
nonfat	½ cup	0
Ices, Sherbets, and Sorbets		
all flavors	½ cup	0

Jams, Jellies, Preserves, and Spreads

All jams, jellies, preserves, and fruit spreads contain 0 grams of fat. They derive all of their calories from carbohydrates, principally sugar.

Pastries*

Food	Serving Size	Fat
apple brown Betty, home recipe	1 cup	5
baklava	1⅓ oz	14
charlotte russe, home recipe	4 oz	16.5
cherry cobbler	4 oz	8
cinnamon bun	2 oz	10
reduced fat	2 oz	3
cream puff, custard filled, home recipe	1 puff; approx 4½ oz	20.25

*Average fat; fat counts vary widely among brands and recipes.

Food	Serving Size	Fat
Pastries *(continued)*		
croissant		
plain, butter, small	1½ oz	10
large	2½ oz	18
almond	3½ oz	25
apple	3½ oz	10
chocolate	3½ oz	24
danish		
cheese	2½ oz	15.5
cinnamon	2½ oz	15
fruit	2½ oz	13
nut	2 oz	16.5
donut		
cake type	1	10.75
chocolate coated	1	13.25
sugared, glazed	1	10.25
jelly filled	1	9.5
holes	5 pieces; 2 oz	10
cruller, glazed	1	7.5
yeast type		
glazed	1	13.75
cream filled	1	20.75
jelly filled	1	16
éclair, custard filled, chocolate iced	3½ oz	14
strudel	2½ oz	8
sweet bun/roll (refrigerated)		
cheese	2 oz	12

Food	Serving Size	Fat
Pastries* *(continued)*		
sweet bun/roll (refrigerated) *(continued)*		
cinnamon raisin	2 oz	10
cinnamon, iced	1½ oz	7
raisin nut	2 oz	7.25
toaster tarts		
apple cinnamon	1¾ oz	5
low fat	1¾ oz	3
blueberry	1¾ oz	5
low fat	1¾ oz	3
brown sugar cinnamon	1¾ oz	7
low fat	1¾ oz	2.75
cherry	1¾ oz	5
low fat	1¾ oz	3
chocolate	1¾ oz	5
low fat	1¾ oz	3
strawberry	1¾ oz	5
low fat	1¾ oz	3
turnover		
apple	2 oz	8
blueberry	2 oz	8
cherry	2 oz	8
Pies and Pie Fillings*		
apple		
pie	⅛ 9" pie	19.5
filling	21 oz can	1

*Average fat; fat counts vary widely among brands and recipes. Pies are per serving; fillings are amount to fill an average pie.

Food	Serving Size	Fat
Pies and Pie Fillings *(continued)*		
banana cream	1/8 9" pie	20
blackberry		
pie	1/8 9" pie	17.5
filling	21 oz can	0
blueberry		
pie	1/8 9" pie	17.5
filling	21 oz can	0
butterscotch		
pie	1/8 9" pie	18.25
filling (see *Puddings and Gelatin*)		
cherry		
pie	1/8 9" pie	22
filling	21 oz can	1
chocolate cream		
pie	1/8 9" pie	23
filling (see *Puddings and Gelatin*)		
chocolate mousse	1/8 9" pie	14.5
coconut cream		
pie	1/8 9" pie	21.25
filling	20 oz can	15
coconut custard	1/6 8" pie	13.75
egg custard	1/6 8" pie	13.25

Food	Serving Size	Fat
Pies and Pie Fillings *(continued)*		
key lime	1/5 8" pie	14
lemon		
pie	1/4 8" pie	15
filling (see *Puddings and Gelatin*)		
meringue	1/8 9" pie	16.5
mincemeat		
pie	1/8 9" pie	17.75
filling	21 oz can	5
peach		
pie	1/8 9" pie	12.5
filling	21 oz can	0
pecan	1/8 9" pie	27
pineapple		
chiffon	1/8 9" pie	9.75
custard	1/8 9" pie	10
pumpkin		
pie	1/8 9" pie	14.5
filling	21 oz can	1
rhubarb	1/8 9" pie	12.5
strawberry		
pie	1/8 9" pie	7.25
strawberry rhubarb	1/6 8" pie	11
filling	21 oz can	0

Food	Serving Size	Fat
Pies and Pie Fillings *(continued)*		
sweet potato	1/8 9" pie	13
vanilla cream		
pie	1/8 9" pie	18
filling (see *Puddings and Gelatin*)		
Pie Crusts and Shells*		
plain		
home recipe	9"	64
made from mix	9"	49
frozen	9"	41.5
graham cracker	9"	40
phyllo	1 sheet	1
puff		
sheet	9 oz	66
shell	1 shell; approx 1½ oz	13
Puddings and Gelatin*		
banana		
made from mix		
with whole milk	½ cup	4.2
with low fat milk	½ cup	2.4
ready to eat	5 oz	5

*Average fat; fat counts vary widely among brands and recipes.

Food	Serving Size	Fat
Puddings and Gelatin *(continued)*		
blancmange, home recipe	½ cup	5
bread, home recipe	½ cup	7.5
butterscotch, ready to eat	4 oz	5.5
chocolate		
home recipe		
with whole milk	½ cup	5.75
with low fat milk	½ cup	4
made from mix		
with whole milk	½ cup	4.75
with low fat milk	½ cup	2.75
ready to eat	5 oz	5.75
fat free	4 oz	.25
coconut cream		
made from mix		
with whole milk	½ cup	5.25
with low fat milk	½ cup	3.5
crème brûlée, home recipe	½ cup	35
crème caramel		
home recipe	½ cup	6.25
made from mix		
with whole milk	½ cup	4
with low fat milk	½ cup	2.5
custard		
baked, home recipe	½ cup	6.5

Food	Serving Size	Fat
Puddings and Gelatin *(continued)*		
custard *(continued)*		
made from mix		
with whole milk	½ cup	5.5
with low fat milk	½ cup	3.75
ready to eat	4 oz	5.25
flan		
home recipe	½ cup	6.25
made from mix		
with whole milk	½ cup	4
with low fat milk	½ cup	2.5
gelatin (made from mix)		
all flavors, regular	½ cup	0
all flavors, artificially sweetened	½ cup	0
lemon		
made from mix		
with whole milk	½ cup	4.25
with sugar, egg yolk, water	½ cup	2
ready to eat	5 oz	4.25
mousse, chocolate		
home recipe	½ cup	33
made from mix	½ cup	5
prune whip, home recipe	1 cup	.25
rice		
home recipe	½ cup	4.25

Food	Serving Size	Fat
Puddings and Gelatin *(continued)*		
rice *(continued)*		
made from mix		
with whole milk	½ cup	4
with low fat milk	½ cup	2.25
ready to eat	5 oz	10.5
tapioca		
home recipe	½ cup	6.5
made from mix		
with whole milk	½ cup	4
with low fat milk	½ cup	2.5
ready to eat	5 oz	5.25
vanilla		
home recipe	½ cup	4
made from mix		
with whole milk	½ cup	4
with low fat milk	½ cup	2.5
ready to eat	½ cup	4
Sauces and Toppings*		
butterscotch	2 tbsp	1.5
caramel	2 tbsp	0
fat free	2 tbsp	0
chocolate		
fudge	2 tbsp	5.75
hot fudge type	2 tbsp	4.25

*Average fat; fat counts vary widely among brands and recipes.

Food	Serving Size	Fat

Sauces and Toppings *(continued)*

chocolate *(continued)*		
mint, fat free	2 tbsp	.5
syrup	2 tbsp	.25
light	2 tbsp	tr
topping	2 tbsp	0
marshmallow cream	2 tbsp	0
pineapple	2 tbsp	0
strawberry	2 tbsp	0
walnut syrup	2 tbsp	9

Sugars, Sweeteners, and Syrups

All sugars, sweeteners, and syrups have 0 fat. They derive all of their calories from sugar, a carbohydrate. These include: **corn syrup, honey, maple syrup, molasses, pancake and waffle syrup, sorghum syrup, sugar, and all artificial sweeteners and sugar substitutes.**

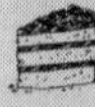

Food	Serving Size	Fat
Vegetables		
alfalfa sprouts	1 cup	.25
artichoke		
whole	10 oz	.5
hearts	1 oz	0
hearts, marinated	1 oz	2
Jerusalem (see *Jerusalem artichoke*)		
arugula	½ cup; approx ⅓ oz	tr
asparagus		
fresh	6 spears; approx 3 oz	.25
canned	½ cup	.75
frozen	4 spears; approx 2 oz	.25
avocado		
California	1	30
Florida	1	27
purée	1 cup	35.25
slices	1 cup	22.25
dip, guacamole (see *Snack Foods*)		
bamboo shoots, canned	1 cup	.5
bean sprouts, mung, raw	½ cup; approx 2 oz	tr

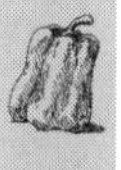

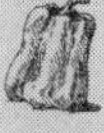

Food	Serving Size	Fat
Vegetables *(continued)*		
beets		
root		
whole, fresh, boiled	3 oz	.25
canned	½ cup; approx 3 oz	tr
pickled	½ cup; approx 4 oz	tr
greens, boiled	½ cup	tr
bell pepper (see *pepper*)		
bok choy		
raw	½ cup; approx 1 oz	tr
cooked	½ cup; approx 3 oz	tr
broccoli		
fresh, raw	1½ oz	.25
fresh, boiled	2¾ oz	.25
frozen, chopped, boiled	½ cup; approx 3¼ oz	tr
Brussels sprouts, boiled	½ cup; approx 2¾ oz	.5
cabbage		
Chinese, raw	½ cup, shredded	tr
green		
raw	½ cup, shredded	tr
boiled	½ cup, shredded	.25

Food	Serving Size	Fat
Vegetables *(continued)*		
cabbage *(continued)*		
red		
raw	½ cup, shredded	tr
boiled	½ cup, shredded	.25
sweet and sour pickled	½ cup	0
Savoy (see *cabbage, green*)		
cole slaw	½ cup	1.5
capers	1 tbsp	0
carrot		
fresh, raw	1 medium; approx 2½ oz	tr
boiled	½ cup, slices	tr
canned	½ cup	tr
frozen	½ cup	tr
dried	1 oz	tr
cassava, raw	3½ oz	.5
cauliflower, fresh, frozen	½ cup, florets	.25
celery	1 stalk	tr
celery root (celeriac), raw	3½ oz	.25
chard (see *Swiss chard*)		
chicory	½ cup; approx 3 oz	.25

Food	Serving Size	Fat
Vegetables *(continued)*		
chives, chopped	1 oz	tr
chiles (see *peppers*)		
collards, chopped, boiled	1 cup; approx 4½ oz	.25
corn		
fresh		
on the cob	5½ oz, with cob	1
kernels	½ cup	1
canned		
in water	½ cup	.75
cream style	½ cup	.5
frozen	½ cup	.5
hominy, canned	1 cup	1.5
cucumber	½ cup slices; approx 2 oz	tr
eggplant, raw	½ cup	tr
endive (chicory, whitloof)	½ cup	0
fennel, bulb, raw	1 cup, slices; approx 3 oz	.25
garlic		
fresh, raw	1 clove	0
chopped, in oil	1 tsp	1
powder	1 tsp	0

Food	Serving Size	Fat
Vegetables *(continued)*		
ginger		
root, fresh	1 oz	.25
root, pickled	1 oz	tr
powder	1 tsp	tr
green beans		
fresh, raw	½ cup	tr
boiled	½ cup; approx 2 oz	.25
canned	½ cup; approx 2 oz	tr
frozen	½ cup; approx 3 oz	.25
green onions (see *scallions*)		
Jerusalem artichoke (sunchoke)	½ cup, slices	0
kale, chopped, boiled	½ cup	.25
leek, chopped	¼ cup; approx 1 oz	tr
lentil sprouts, raw	½ cup	.25
lettuce, all types	½ oz, shredded; 1 oz	tr
lima beans		
fresh, boiled	½ cup	.25
canned	½ cup	.25

Food	Serving Size	Fat
Vegetables *(continued)*		
lima beans *(continued)*		
frozen	½ cup	.25
dried *(see Beans)*		
mixed vegetables		
frozen	½ cup	0
canned	½ cup	0
mung bean, sprouts (*see bean sprouts*)		
mushrooms		
fresh, raw	½ cup; approx 1 oz	0
canned	½ cup; approx 3 oz	.25
dried (shiitake)	1 oz	tr
mustard greens, boiled	½ cup, chopped	.25
okra		
raw	½ cup; approx 2 oz	tr
boiled	½ cup; approx 3 oz	.25
olives		
all types, small–large	1 olive	.5
all types, jumbo–colossal	1 olive	1
oil cured	1 oz; approx 10 olives	7

Food	Serving Size	Fat
Vegetables *(continued)*		
onion		
fresh, raw	3 oz	tr
small, frozen	½ cup; 4 oz	tr
dried, flakes	¼ cup; ½ oz	tr
fried rings, battered	2 oz	7
pickled, cocktail	1 tbsp	0
green (see *scallions*)		
palm, hearts	1 oz	.25
parsley		
fresh	½ cup, chopped	.25
dried	¼ tsp	0
freeze dried	1 tsp	tr
root	1 oz	.5
parsnip, raw or cooked	½ cup, slices	.25
pea pods (see *snow peas*)		
peas, black-eye (see *Beans*)		
peas, green		
fresh, raw, shelled	½ cup	.25
frozen	½ cup	.25
canned, all types	½ cup	.25

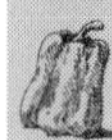
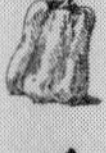
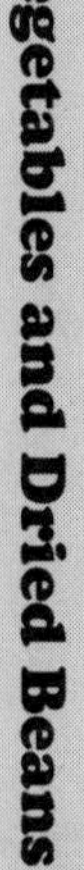
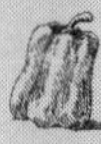

Food	Serving Size	Fat
Vegetables *(continued)*		
pepper		
hot, chile		
raw	1½ oz	tr
green, canned	¼ cup	tr
jalapeno, diced, canned	2 tbsp	.25
sweet, green, red, yellow		
raw, whole	medium	tr
raw, chopped	½ cup	tr
frozen	1 cup	0
roasted	1 oz	0
roasted, in olive oil	1 oz	1
pimiento	1 tbsp	0
cherry, pickled	1 oz	0
plantain (see *Fruits)*		
pickles, all types	1 oz	0
potato		
fresh, raw, without skin	4 oz	tr
diced, peeled	1 cup	tr
canned, without skin	½ cup	.25
baked, microwaved, with skin	7 oz	.25
boiled	4 oz	tr
au gratin	½ cup	9.25
fried, pan	3 oz	15
French-fried	2 oz	10
hash brown	½ cup	10
mashed		
home recipe, with milk and butter	½ cup	4
instant	½ cup	6

Food	Serving Size	Fat
Vegetables *(continued)*		
potato *(continued)*		
kugel	5 oz	20
pancake	1 oz	5
salad		
German style	½ cup	3
with mayo	½ cup	10.25
scalloped	½ cup	4.5
sweet (see *sweet potato*)		
pumpkin, canned, unsweetened	½ cup	.25
pie mix (see *Sweets and Desserts: Pie Fillings*)		
radicchio	½ cup, shredded	tr
radish	1 oz	tr
rhubarb	½ cup	tr
rutabaga, boiled	½ cup, cubes	.25
sauerkraut	½ cup	0
sweet and sour	½ cup	0
scallions	½ cup, chopped	tr
shallot	1 tbsp, chopped	0
snow peas		
raw	3 oz	0
boiled	½ cup	.25

Food	Serving Size	Fat
Vegetables *(continued)*		
snow peas *(continued)*		
frozen	3 oz	1.5
soybeans, fresh		
boiled	½ cup	5.75
sprouts	1 cup	6
soybean products		
soy flour *(see Sweets and Desserts: Baking Ingredients)*		
soy milk, tofu *(see Diet and Health Foods)*		
soy sauce, miso *(see Extras)*		
soynuts *(see Nuts and Seeds)*		
spinach		
fresh, raw	½ cup, chopped	tr
canned, frozen	½ cup	tr
creamed	½ cup	2
sprouts (see *individual vegetable*)		
squash		
summer: zucchini, yellow		
raw	½ cup, sliced	tr
boiled	½ cup	.25
winter: acorn, butternut, hubbard		
raw	½ cup, cubes	tr
baked	½ cup, cubes	.5
boiled, mashed	½ cup	tr

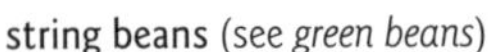

string beans (see *green beans*)

Food	Serving Size	Fat
Vegetables *(continued)*		
sugar snap peas (see *snow peas*)		
sunchoke (see *Jerusalem artichoke*)		
sweet potato		
raw	4 oz	.5
baked, steamed	4 oz	tr
mashed	1 cup	.5
candied	3¾ oz	3.5
canned		
in light syrup	½ cup; 4 oz	.25
in heavy syrup	½ cup; 4½ oz	0
chips (see *Snack Foods: Chips*)		
Swiss chard, boiled	½ cup, chopped	tr
tomatillo, raw	1 medium; approx 1 oz	.25
tomato		
fresh, raw	1 medium; approx 4 oz	.5
green	1 medium; approx 4 oz	.25
boiled	½ cup	.5
canned		
paste	2 tbsp	.5
purée	1 cup	.5
stewed	1 cup	2
whole, peeled	1 cup	.5

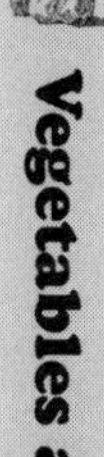
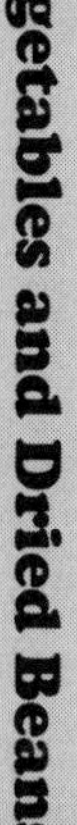

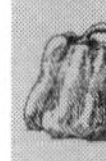

Food	Serving Size	Fat
Vegetables *(continued)*		
tomato *(continued)*		
sun dried	2 oz	2.5
in oil	1 cup	15.5
turnip, raw	½ cup	tr
water chestnuts, canned	½ cup	0
watercress	1 cup; 1 oz	0
yam (see *sweet potato*)		
zucchini (see *squash, summer*)		
Beans (dried, legumes)		
adzuki		
boiled	1 cup	.25
canned, sweetened	1 cup	tr
baked*	1 cup	13
black		
dried, uncooked	½ cup	.75
boiled	½ cup	.5
canned	½ cup	1
sauce (see *Extras: Sauces*)		

*Average fat; fat count and serving size vary widely among brands.

Food	Serving Size	Fat
Beans (dried, legumes) *(continued)*		
black-eye peas		
fresh, raw	½ cup	.25
boiled	½ cup	.25
dried	½ cup	1.5
boiled	½ cup	0
canned	½ cup	1
broad		
boiled	1 cup	.75
canned	1 cup	.5
chickpeas (garbanzo beans)		
dried, uncooked	¼ cup	2
boiled	1 cup	4.5
canned	1 cup	2.75
hummus (see *Snack Foods: Dips*)		
cow peas (see *black-eye peas*)		
cranberry beans		
dried, uncooked	½ cup	.75
boiled	1 cup	.75
canned	1 cup	.75
garbanzo (see *chickpeas*)		
great northern		
dried, uncooked	½ cup	.75
boiled	1 cup	.75
canned	1 cup	1

Food	Serving Size	Fat
Beans (dried, legumes) *(continued)*		
kidney		
dried, uncooked	½ cup	1.5
boiled	1 cup	1
canned	1 cup	.75
lentils		
dried, uncooked	½ cup	0
boiled	1 cup	.5
sprouts (see *Vegetables*)		
lima		
fresh (see *Vegetables*)		
dried, uncooked	½ cup	1.5
boiled	1 cup	0
navy		
dried, uncooked	½ cup	1.5
boiled	1 cup	1
canned	1 cup	1
peas, split		
dried, uncooked	½ cup	.5
boiled	1 cup	.75
pinto		
dried, uncooked	½ cup	1.5
boiled	1 cup	1
canned	1 cup	2